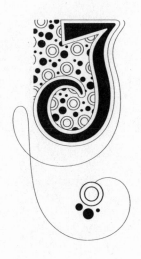

NATURALLY

HOW TO LOOK AND FEEL
HEALTHY, ENERGETIC AND RADIANT
THE ORGANIC WAY

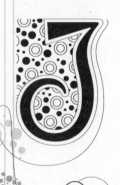

JO WOOD

with Jane Ross-Macdonald

SIDGWICK & JACKSON

First published 2007 by Sidgwick & Jackson
an imprint of Pan Macmillan Ltd
Pan Macmillan, 20 New Wharf Road, London N1 9RR
Basingstoke and Oxford
Associated companies throughout the world
www.panmacmillan.com

ISBN 978-0-283-07041-9

3 5 7 9 8 6 4 2

A CIP catalogue record for this book is available from
the British Library.

Printed and bound in Great Britain by
Mackays of Chatham plc, Chatham, Kent

Visit www.panmacmillan.com to read more about all our books
and to buy them. You will also find features, author interviews and
news of any author events, and you can sign up for e-newsletters
so that you're always first to hear about our new releases.

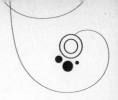

For my mother, my husband, children,
brothers and sisters, who have all given me
so much love, creativity and laughter.

In loving memory of my father,
Michael Karslake and absent loved ones.

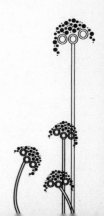

Acknowledgements

I'd like to thank Gerald Green, who started me on my organic journey, Dr Nish Joshi, who allowed us to reproduce his food list from Dr Joshi's Holistic Detox, Jeff Hewitt from Hewitt Landscapes and Patrick Harty from Sandymount, who helped with the gardening section, Jenny Taylor from Holmwood, Renée Elliot from Planet Organic for letting me use their lovely juice recipes, Tina Abbey from Holistic Touch, who supplied the text on yoga, Mike Doxey who helps me train, Dr Colette Haydon for her help with chapter 7 and Franzesca Watson for advising on the aromatherapy section.

I have to thank family and friends for their contribution: my husband Ronnie, our children, Jamie, Jesse, Leah and Tyrone; my mum, Rachel Karslake; sister, Lize McCarron; and brothers, Paul and Vini Karslake. Keith Richards and Patti Hansen Richards, Mick Jagger, Charlie Watts, Cilla Black, Patrick Holden, William and Gaby Lana, who all gave me quotes. Jamie Oliver and Josephine Fairley Sams for their inspiring example.

A big thank you to Emily Harper and Donna Worling, who work with me and keep me sane, Jane Ross-Macdonald for putting my thoughts into words, to my editor Ingrid Connell and agent Pat Lomax. To Amy Rowe for helping with the research and Annie Rigg for casting an eagle eye over the recipes.

And thanks to The Nest, for making my products look so sophisticated and beautiful, and for the illustrative motifs used in this book.

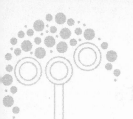

Contents

Introduction

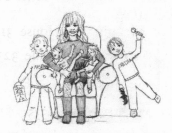

My name is Josephine Wood and I am a self-confessed organic nut. I'm also wife to my famous husband, Ronnie, mother to four wonderful grown-up kids – Jamie, Jesse, Leah and Ty – and granny to four wonderful grandchildren. I have had a great life: I have travelled the world, watched my husband play to millions, met lots of interesting people, seen wonderful places. I have been very lucky. My mother always said, 'Better to be born lucky than rich,' and she was right. Some people call me a rock chick, but I prefer the term 'chic nomad'.

Since my conversion from someone whose mantra used to be 'pass me the ciggies' to 'who wants an organic beetroot juice?',

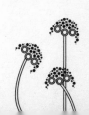

Introduction

I have delved more and more deeply into what it really means to be organic – what a healthy, natural lifestyle entails, not just in terms of shopping and gardening, but in the kinds of food you put into your body, what you surround yourself with, and how you treat your body and the world around you. I still love to party, but now I feel more grounded.

In this book I'll show you a little of what I have learnt along the way about how to live in tune with yourself and the natural environment. You'll find tips on living organically, delicious recipes, ideas for growing your own fruit and vegetables, my own beauty secrets and lots of my favourite ways to relax and feel good. Above all, it's about finding your own path in life and living as well as you can.

I hope you will feel sufficiently inspired to try some of the ideas I suggest for yourself.

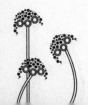

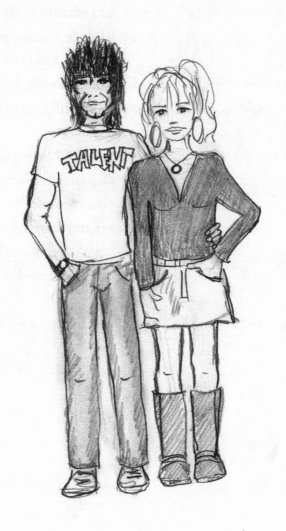
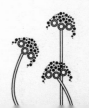

'Josephine's preoccupation with organic food, people's health and helping save the planet has almost reached obsession pitch. What my wife says is well researched, full of truth and usually extremely beneficial to the body, the mind and general well-being. Read what she says with an open mind and you will find it helpful to both you and friends in need. I am very proud of her advances towards a healthier you and a safer planet.'

Ronnie Wood

Part I

Eating Organically

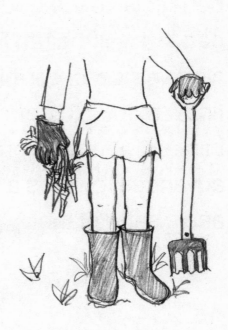

Jo's been in a bit of a panic

Her task is tough and titanic

The opposition is dark and satanic

Their methods are cruel and barbaric

So she's gone completely organic

While she's trying to rescue the planet

So go buy this book – goddamit!!

Mick Jagger

I

Finding Shangri-La

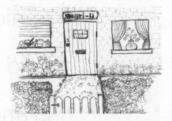

MY CONVERSION TO ORGANIC LIVING, which occurred when it was still pretty unfashionable, was sparked by a life-changing event. At the time, Ronnie and I had been together for about fourteen years, and it seemed as if my life couldn't get any better – my kids were growing up well-adjusted and loving, plus I had a husband who adored me. There were countless parties, lots of late nights and wonderful days. One night in 1989, though, just after we'd bought a fantastic Georgian house by the canal in County Kildare, Ireland, we went for dinner with friends in Dublin. During the evening, I suddenly felt ill and went outside, where I was violently sick with pains in my stomach like you wouldn't believe. Ronnie tried to help,

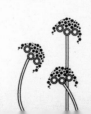

but there was no denying I was really ill, so he insisted I go to the hospital to get checked out. The next day the doctors said they were not sure what it was and wanted to do more tests. By now, however, I was feeling better and, as I was very keen to go to Morocco (where the Stones were recording), off I went. I was fine on that trip, but when I got home I was sick again. This time I was diagnosed with Crohn's disease (an inflammation of the intestine) and put on two kinds of steroids – yuck. They took my spirit away. I went to see four doctors, in the hope of being told something different, but they all said the same thing: Crohn's disease.

So I began to live with it, all the time believing I would one day find a cure. I didn't know how or where I would find it, but I always had an open mind and was willing to try anything that came along.

About a year later, I got a request for an interview about my illness. I must admit the headline 'Stone's Wife has Incurable Disease' in huge letters in the tabloid press was not what I had intended. But two weeks later the office rang to say the paper had sent over a big bag full of letters for me. I read them all. One letter in particular struck me. It was from a man called Gerald Greene, a herbalist. In it he told me that if I went to see him he would be able to put my Crohn's disease into remission for life. That was what I had been waiting for! So I asked a girlfriend to come with me and

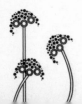

off I went to Hastings. That was the start of my fantastic organic journey.

I wondered if I was on my way to a madman or my saviour when I arrived at a house named Shangri-La. 'Sit down, Jo,' Gerald said gently. I wasn't sure where to sit, as the tiny house was packed with books, bottles, pots and God knows what else. I found a corner of a sofa. After a few moments we were chatting like old friends, and I was giving him what were probably quite intimate details about my digestive system.

'Four doctors have told me I have Crohn's disease,' I finished, looking at him expectantly.

'Yes, my dear. Whatever your disease is, I need to know what it is that you eat.'

This was a surprise. I had never given my diet much thought. I wanted a cure, not to talk about the contents of my fridge.

'Oh, ordinary stuff. Pork chops, frozen peas. Whatever I have to hand – normal supermarket food. I cook a lot of those slimming ready meals. I mix up packet stuff. Sometimes, if I can't be bothered to cook, I eat takeaways, and I love Kentucky Fried Chicken.' He was nodding sagely.

'You've got to change your whole way of eating if you want to get well,' he said after a pause. 'You have a lot to learn.'

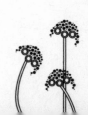

'What do you mean?'

'All of those foods you have mentioned, you will have to stop eating them,' he said simply.

Oh my God. 'Why?'

'It's all to do with your immune system. If you don't look after it, you'll be in trouble.'

I was intrigued. 'Tell me more.'

'Let me describe it to you the way I explain it to my patients. The immune system is like an army. There are generals, officers and private soldiers called lymphocytes. The T-cell lymphocytes are the generals, who give orders to their B-cell officers and private soldiers (called B-cell antibodies) to attack anything bad which attacks the body. Just as in an army, these "soldiers" are split into regiments, with one regiment assigned to each vital part of our bodies, so protecting us from any attacks, from any quarter, any time. Are you following me, my dear?'

'I think so.'

'Now, some people have fragile immune systems, and what happens when they ingest inorganic chemicals from insecticides, fungicides and herbicides in our foods is that the general-like T-cells misprogramme one of the multiple regiments protecting our vital parts, and whatever that regiment was protecting *it now attacks*. This

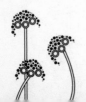

is called an autoimmune disease and includes diseases such as MS, Crohn's, ulcerative colitis, systemic lupus and so on.'

'Caused by chemicals in our diet?'

'I believe so, and I'll come on to these in a moment. But first let me tell you about candida. This is a friendly yeast everyone has (initially at least) and its purpose is to feed the beneficial gut bugs at night while we sleep so that during the day they can do their wonderful digestive work. If, however, the person has a nasty disease that is treated by antibiotics, steroids or chemotherapy, these good bugs are destroyed – so there is nothing left to eat their ever-growing food source: candida. So what happens is that candida grows out of control and turns into a very unfriendly fungus that punctures the bowel wall, sometimes causing an allergic response to foods, which in turn triggers the symptoms of the diseases I have already mentioned.'

'That sounds awful.'

'It is, but to add insult to injury, candida then gets into the bloodstream, where it ingests blood sugar and converts it to alcohol, leading to fatigue. The patient becomes a slave to alcohol: not like a normal alcoholic, but to the "fix" from sugary foods. And so it continues. I have seen patients with Crohn's disease come off sugar and shake as if they have DTs.'

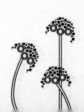

Eating Organically

'Oh my God, it sounds terrible. What can I do?'

'Take it one step at a time, my dear. I specialise in treating autoimmune diseases, of which Crohn's is just one, and I have had extraordinary success. There are three things you must do to start building up your immune system to give your body a chance of fighting back. The first is to change your diet completely, and I'll come on to this. The second is to eat organic food, and the third is to take some of my herbal pills.'

'I'm sorry, I don't know what you mean by organic food.' (This was fifteen years ago, remember.)

'Organic food is food that is grown without the use of chemicals. Of course, all things are made up of chemical compounds, as you probably know, but I'm talking about synthetic chemicals, manmade in a laboratory. Chemicals that prevent your immune system from working properly. Many of the chemicals used on our food today are organophosphates, which started life as nerve gas in the First World War.'

Organic? I had never heard of it, or, to be more accurate, I had heard the word, but had no idea what it meant. Gerald talked for two hours about how food is produced, where it comes from and what is done to it before it gets on to our plates. He talked about things I had never given any thought to – about farming techniques, about soil, about the conditions animals are kept in, and about hormones, pesticides, colourings and flavourings. He was opening up a new world and I was horrified yet fascinated. It all made so much sense. I understood how it was that we had come too far from the natural way of producing and eating food – so far, in fact, that our bodies could not deal with what we were asking them to digest. Our guts had not developed the features necessary to deal with our modern diet, and our livers could not process the poisons quickly or efficiently enough. They stayed in our bodies and made us ill. In addition, certain foodstuffs clogged up the digestive system and stopped the real nutrients getting to the body. Now I understood why the steroids I had been taking had made me feel a whole lot worse.

'Those pills you are taking will kill you before your digestive disease will,' he concluded.

I wanted to know more. I loved what he was telling me and I wanted to get better. This had to be the answer: I was sick of doctors, sick of being ill, and I hung on his every word.

'Yes! You're right. The pills have made my symptoms better, but I just don't feel like myself – and look at me, I look terrible. If I come off them, though, will my stomach pain come back? What can I do?' I pressed him for answers.

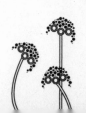

Eating Organically

'You must follow this diet,' he said, handing me some leaflets, 'it will ease your candida problem. And you must gradually come off the steroids. It is important to cleanse your body, and these herbal pills will help. They contain a mixture of natural healing plants: slippery elm, golden seal and liquorice. They will coat your insides so you can eat your new cleansing diet without feeling ill.'

'What is the diet?'

'No wheat or dairy products and no red meat. No processed food. Lots of vegetables, a little fish and chicken, and make sure they are produced without added chemicals. Avoid anything that candida loves – which includes sugar, yeast and carbohydrates. And, as I have explained to you, you must get hold of food that has been produced *organically*.'

What he was suggesting sounded pretty difficult, but I was prepared to try anything. Realising I had been there for hours, I paid him for the herbs, thanked him and said goodbye.

'Stick at it, Jo,' he said as we left. 'As my grandfather used to say, "Only the impossible is difficult; the rest is a piece of cake".'

He stood on his doorstep watching us drive down the lane, an old man full of wisdom and kindness who had reached out to a complete stranger. By now I felt strongly that he wasn't a madman, but just how much of a saviour he would turn out to be I couldn't then have known.

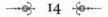

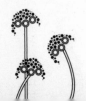

Finding Shangri-La

On the way home I reflected on what he had said. Why had no one ever told me this before? It was so obvious, really, if I thought about it. Our bodies simply were not adapted to the mix of foods, saturated fats, additives and chemicals we were asking them to absorb. Many hundreds of generations had passed since people had had to subsist on a diet of vegetables and nuts, and that kind of diet no longer suited our lifestyles, but now that multinational corporations with slick marketing operations had got involved in the business of mass food production, we had gradually been taken further and further away from what our bodies need. Time had moved on, but the human digestive system hadn't. In order to produce the amount of food consumers wanted crops were being sprayed with chemicals to kill fungi, insects, weeds and bacteria. How could it not be harming both us and the environment? Yet – like millions of other people – I thought it was perfectly fine to exist on a diet of meat and two veg, a bit of fruit here and there, nice puddings, takeaways when I fancied them, and lots of processed convenience foods full of sugar.

I was slowly killing myself, and – let's face it – my busy lifestyle touring the world wasn't exactly helping. I knew I was being offered a golden opportunity. I was sick and tired of feeling sick and tired: Gerald was offering me the chance to live well, and to create a healthier life for my children. I grabbed it with both hands.

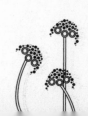

The change in my health was amazing – it was as if my soul had come back. My skin cleared, my hair shone and my eyes sparkled. I was happy and laughing again when, three months after Shangri-La, I had a setback. I was at a friend's house when suddenly I doubled up in pain. It was back – the terrible gut-wrenching agony. I was appalled, angry and shocked. How could this be happening again?

'What's going on?' asked my friend Lorraine in horror. 'I thought you were cured.'

'So did I,' I moaned.

It turned out that my friend's father knew an amazing intestinal specialist called Professor Farthing. Well, I had nothing to lose, I thought, but I was miserable at the prospect of reverting to traditional doctors, and no way was I going back on steroids. I had a consultation with Professor Farthing the very next day, and straightaway he did several tests, including giving me a Barium meal.

'I don't think you've got Crohn's disease,' he said.

'Great.' This was fantastic news – but God, what could it be? Cancer? I asked him what he thought, and he hedged his bets.

'I'm not sure, we'll need to have a look inside you to find out exactly what it is.'

I was terrified. I had never had an operation, and the night before what they were calling 'exploratory surgery' I looked down at

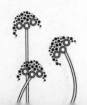

my smooth, flat tummy knowing that the next day it would have a big scar right down the middle.

After the operation we had our answer. I had had a perforated appendix. I must have had it all the time. Because it was infected, it had been inflaming the intestine, which explained why I had been in so much pain and why the doctors thought I had Crohn's disease. Needless to say, they removed it, plus some of my intestine. As I was recovering in the hospital bed, the surgeon came to see me.

'You have had a lucky escape. If you had stayed on the steroids you were given for Crohn's disease they would have continued to mask the symptoms and one of these days the perforated appendix would have burst. That is not something I would wish on anyone. You could have died.'

'What about my new diet?'

'I think it's doing you a great deal of good. Apart from your appendix, the rest of your gut looked pretty healthy to me.'

So I wasn't suffering from an incurable disease after all. I was relieved beyond measure at this diagnosis, but furious with those other supposedly top doctors who had told me I'd had Crohn's, especially because it had led to the terrible year on steroids. But at the same time I recognised that if it hadn't been for the chance contact with Gerald Greene my life would be very different today. He opened my eyes to a new way of living.

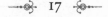

2

An Organic Life

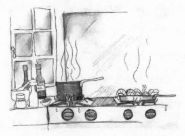

So it was that, fifteen years ago, I chucked out all my non-organic food and started the search for organic products. It was a hard task. None of the supermarkets stocked them, and the selection in the few health food shops I found was not only limited, but also slightly past its best.

I asked our gardener, Patrick, who works for us in County Kildare, to start digging up the flowerbeds and to plant vegetables, but it would be some time before these were ready. When they were, I used to transport heavy suitcases of potatoes back to London on the plane. In the end, I found someone who would bring me a big box of fresh fruit and vegetables from an organic farm, and when that happened

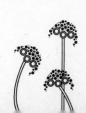

I started in earnest. I was like a woman possessed, and everywhere I went I demanded organic produce. When I did manage to get hold of it, it was a revelation. For not only was organic food healthier, it was actually much tastier than non-organic food. I had been expecting food just like what I had been used to, but without chemicals, yet here I was discovering new delicious tastes! I had grown used to pepping up bland food with ketchup, salt, butter and various sauces; now I liked my vegetables *au naturel* – because at last they tasted like themselves. Why was this? I wondered. What exactly did 'organic' mean? Why was it important? I just had the few leaflets that Gerald had given me, but I wanted more, so I set about reading as much as I could about what I was fast realising was a strong grass-roots movement.

In those days, information was pretty hard to come by. I haunted my local health food shop, and drove all over the country looking for others. I picked up leaflets and buried myself in obscure books published by small cooperatives. No one I knew was talking about organic food, and no one seemed interested. It became a passion, though, and I would lecture my friends and family, and probably – looking back – got pretty boring about it. Like millions of people, I had taken for granted what I was putting into my mouth, but, once I started to question it, I knew everyone had to know about what I now knew. I preached, I lectured, and at first people switched off.

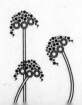

An Organic Life

When I visited LA in the early 1990s, a friend told me to go to a small organic supermarket off Rodeo Drive. When I walked in, I thought I'd died and gone to heaven. They had organic toothpaste, organic deodorant, T-shirts, bath stuff, tampons, everything. It was all pure – it was fantastic, I just couldn't believe it, I wanted to bring the whole thing back to England. If they could do it, why couldn't we have something like that over here? This was what I had been searching for. It was unbelievable. I spent hours and hours there and came back with hundreds of paper bags of stuff I didn't know even existed. After that, things seemed to happen quite quickly – Planet Organic and Fresh and Wild started up, and, at the same time, I found people began to sit up and take notice. I started meeting more like-minded people and, over time, got invited to attend the Organic Food Awards.

So this is what I would tell anyone who would listen. The way our world deals with the food we eat has changed dramatically over the past century. Whereas not so long ago we would have eaten food that had been grown and stored close to our homes, now half the planet's population of six billion people live in cities and do not grow their own food. Non-organic crops are planted in the same fields year after year (a system known as 'monoculture'), which means the soil loses essential nutrients as it is gradually stripped of its nutritional

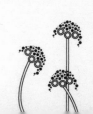

goodness. It is therefore enriched with nitrogenous fertilisers, some of which washes into rivers, lakes and aquifers, polluting them, reducing the oxygen levels in the water and threatening wildlife. This nitrogen has to be removed from drinking water – and the cost ultimately is passed on to the public.

THE EFFECTS OF MONOCULTURE

Non-organic, monoculture crops are sprayed with chemical fertilisers to encourage fast growth and more frequent harvesting, resulting in greater profits for farmers. The industrial processes used to produce these chemical fertilisers, however, use up valuable energy. And because the soil lacks nutrients, the plants grown in it lack nutrients too, with the result that they are more open to attack by pests and diseases. To combat this, non-organic food is also sprayed with fungicides, pesticides and herbicides to kill mould, insects and small animals and weeds. This stuff is POISONOUS – and it stays on the food that we eat, however much we wash it. The birds and insects that feed on these pests and weeds are denied their food source – which means the whole ecosystem is affected. In addition:

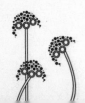

☠ Meat and dairy products come from animals that are fed cheap, non-organic feed. These animals are given extra vitamins to compensate for the lack of nutrition in their feed, plus hormones to encourage faster growth. They are also routinely given antibiotics (even if they are not sick) to keep them disease-free and to fatten them up.

☠ There is evidence that this over-use of antibiotics creates superbugs, bacteria resistant to the common antibiotics.

☠ Diseases such as mad cow disease and salmonella spread because the farmers' need to produce more and more food more cheaply became more important to them than the welfare of their animals. Even now there are millions of cases of salmonella and E. coli reported annually worldwide.

Since monoculture was introduced in the 1940s, the incidence of autoimmune diseases such as Crohn's, ulcerative colitis, multiple sclerosis and so on has gone through the roof. Ironically, the pharmaceutical products used to control these diseases are often made by the same companies that market the deadly crop chemicals.

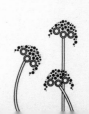

Eating Organically

Another side effect of monoculture is that many varieties of fruit and vegetables are simply not grown any more because they are unprofitable. Where once the UK had 6,000 varieties of apples, now it is hard to find more than a dozen in the supermarkets.

Organic farmers on the other hand:

- Use natural fertilisers which, though slower-acting, do not run off and damage our soil and water systems.

- Use animal manure and plant wastes as natural compost.

- Weed mechanically rather than spraying.

- Rotate crops to allow the soil to recover its natural fertility and to reduce the risk of crop diseases building up in the soil.

- Have higher standards of animal welfare – animals are kept in more natural, free-range conditions and eat a more natural diet. Drugs and antibiotics are not used routinely.

- Do not grow GM crops and can only, as a last resort, use seven of the many hundreds of pesticides.

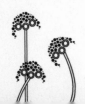

Organic farms and food companies are inspected at least once a year and to be certified organic they must meet the criteria set out by the regulating bodies in their country. There are a number of different certification bodies in the UK, but they all stick to the basic standards set by DEFRA (the Department for Environment, Food and Rural Affairs). The Soil Association certifies about 75 per cent of UK produce. In Europe the basic standards are set by IFOAM (the International Federation for Organic Agriculture Movements). Under the strict guidelines laid down by certifying bodies such as the Soil Association, organic farming encourages the flourishing of the natural ecosystem and lower carbon dioxide emissions. Organic food, crucially, avoids over 400 pesticides and additives.

What Pesticides Do to Us

Just in case you're sitting there thinking, pesticides – huh – how bad can they be? Here's what happens. Even if each apple, pear or carrot contains a lower than legally permitted amount of pesticide residue (and not all of them do), these tiny amounts build up in your body over time. Scientists have found residues from more than fifty pesticides on conventionally grown (i.e. non-organic) food. The

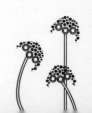

safety testing of pesticides assumes healthy adults; it does not take into account the very old, the very young, or adolescents who may be vulnerable and whose hormonal systems are changing.

While we're at it, let's give them their names. It's helpful to know your enemy, after all, and one day perhaps food will be properly labelled. The substances we are talking about include Chlorpropham, Folpet, Carbendazim, Chorpyrifos, Lindane, Chlormequat, Vinclozalin and organophosphates. Many of them cannot be got rid of by washing and peeling, although that helps a little. Laboratory research has indicated – although the jury is still out – that these substances are variously linked with cancer, birth defects, nerve damage, behavioural disorders, early puberty and infertility, not to mention the autoimmune problems first explained to me by Gerald Greene. Personally, I'm not prepared to wait until the jury returns its verdict, particularly as it is the long-term build up of these chemicals that concerns me.

As adults, our bodies may be better at resisting this onslaught, but children are different. Their internal organs are still developing, and in relation to their body weight they actually eat and drink more than adults, thereby increasing their exposure. They may even (let's hope so, anyway) eat more fruit and vegetables than we do. Pesticides may block the absorption of important nutrients children need for

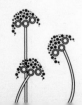

healthy growth. It is thought that babies may absorb pesticides more easily and break them down less easily. Isn't this terrible? You encourage your children to eat their 'five a day' and – because there is no law obliging producers and manufacturers to tell us what pesticides have been sprayed on our food – you are actually force-feeding them these harmful substances.

PROCESSED FOODS

Processed foods have been blamed for the large rise in obesity and chronic disease levels around the world as they are high in saturated fats (including the most unhealthy, hydrogenated fat), sugar and salt. Processed foods are also full of additives, including artificial colourings and flavourings (often, but not always, described as E numbers), which have been found to cause health problems such as migraines, hyperactivity, allergies, asthma, osteoporosis and heart disease. Frankly, there's now so much research around that I can't understand why they are permitted any more.

I know that sometimes we just don't have time to cook a meal from scratch, but at least these days it is possible to find organic processed food. Organic processed food contains far fewer additives – the EU

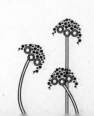

allows only 35, compared to the over 500 that can be used in non-organic food, and the Soil Association has reduced this list further on foods it certifies. Additives in organic food are generally derived from natural sources and don't include artificial colourings or flavourings, but the quality can vary, depending on the manufacturer, and it can still be high in fat, sugar and salt – you really need to read the label of any processed food before you buy it.

ORGANIC BABY FOOD

Although it's definitely best to give your baby food you've cooked yourself, in reality there can't be many parents who haven't bought the ready-made version. While there are strict guidelines about what is allowed in non-organic baby food – no preservatives or artificial colouring, for example – they can contain starches and more water than is necessary to bulk them out. More importantly, you can't be sure that the food itself isn't contaminated with agrochemicals or antibiotics. Babies up to the age of one are particularly vulnerable to toxins, as their immune system, nervous system, liver and kidneys are so immature. It makes sense to choose organic baby food as you know the raw ingredients aren't contaminated in this way. As ever

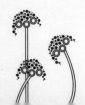

with processed food, check that it is really organic and always read the label, as some of the bigger manufacturers have leapt on to the organic bandwagon and may include ingredients that aren't harmful (water, for example) but which you may not expect to see.

'I've always been fascinated by Jo's passion for all things organic. She truly does believe we can change the world, and help the environment if we all go organic. I must admit I agree with her, having grown all my own vegetables since the 1970s. It truly is the way to go.'

Cilla Black

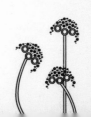

Eating Organically

CHOOSING ORGANIC

You can now find organic food in health food shops, most supermarkets, specialist chains, farm shops and farmers markets. You can also sign up for a box delivery scheme. You've got to try not to mind if your food arrives covered in mud, looks a bit dull or is oddly shaped – it tastes much better! My friend Lorraine once called late at night and said she was coming over, and was *starving*. I pulled on my wellies, headed for the vegetable patch, and picked some lettuce, tomatoes and cucumber for her by the light of the full moon. There was something magical about that meal, and Lorraine declared it to be the most delicious salad she had ever tasted.

I conducted an experiment once, too. I was going away for a month and left some non-organic tomatoes in the fridge. I made sure no one touched them in my absence, and when I came back they were still fresh, preserved by all the chemicals – how scary.

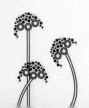

Box Schemes

Thankfully there are now some wonderful companies and cooperatives that will bring fresh organic produce direct to your door from farms. Not just vegetables and fruit, but cheese, meat, eggs, fish, wine and cleaning products. You can sign up for a weekly 'family box' or be more specific each week about your choices. You'll find lovely seasonal stuff, and it means you don't need to think about what to cook – just make your mind up when it arrives! Some of them even come with recipe suggestions. Check the internet for your local organic box schemes or see the resource section at the back of this book.

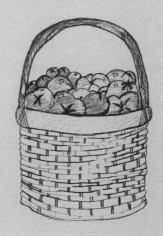

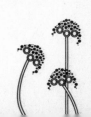

Eating Organically

The only downside to converting to organic everything is the price-tag. It is more expensive, but I just believe it's worth it. Having been ill, I learnt first-hand that health is the greatest gift we have. I know some people will think that it's all very well for her, she can afford it, and you'd be right, I can. I do think, though, that if we all took a stand against the use of the chemicals that are making us and our children sick, the food production in this country would have to improve, and organic food would get cheaper. At the moment it's expensive because organic farms produce smaller crops and need to work harder producing them.

I know we've got to be realistic here, and I accept that not only do we sometimes shop in a rush, but that often we can't find the organic version of what we're looking for. When this happens, it is as well to remember that there are some foods that absorb pesticides more readily than others. These are:

Apples

Bananas

Breakfast cereals

Carrots

Celery

Cherries

Dried fruits

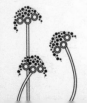

An Organic Life

Foods containing animal fats (e.g. cheese, butter, milk)

Grapes

Lettuces

Nectarines

Peaches

Peanuts

Pears

Peppers

Potatoes

Raspberries

Rice

Spinach

Strawberries

If you can, select an alternative from the following list, as these fruits and vegetables tend to absorb fewer pollutants:

Asparagus

Avocados

Broccoli

Cabbage

Cauliflower

Kiwi

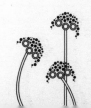

Eating Organically

Mangoes
Onions
Papaya
Peas
Pineapples
Sweetcorn

If you do end up buying non-organic food make sure you:

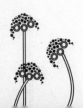 Peel it, or remove the outer leaves of vegetables such as cabbage and lettuce.

Wash those you don't peel, using a produce wash product such as Citrus Magic Veggie Spray, available from *www.veggie-wash.com*.

Choose a wide variety of products to prevent the build up of just one or two pesticides.

Trim the fat and skin off poultry (organocholoride pesticides tend to be stored in animal fat).

And if you are still unconvinced as to why it's best to choose organic, here are a few more reasons:

Cheese ᴣ A build up of antibiotics from the milk used to make non-organic cheese makes you more susceptible to infections. Imported non-organic cheese has been found to contain the poison lindane.

Fruit and vegetables ᴣ If they are organic, you don't have to worry about residues from pesticides, herbicides, etc., which means you can eat the skin too (good for increasing your fibre intake and sometimes the highest concentration of vitamins is just under the skin). Plus they contain more nutrients because of the nutrient-rich soil they have been grown in.

Milk ᴣ Organic milk contains no antibiotics, fertility hormones or chemical residues and has higher levels of the essential fatty acid Omega 3, vitamin E and antioxidants.

Oats ᴣ Organic oats are richer in B vitamins, better for the nervous system.

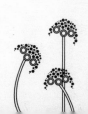

Eating Organically

Potatoes ॐ Organic potatoes contain far more zinc and potassium than their non-organic rivals, which are doused in chemicals about ten times during the growing period and even sprayed after picking to prolong their shelf life.

Eggs ॐ If the eggs are labelled free range it means they come from chickens that will not have suffered in battery farms. All organic eggs are free range; in addition, the Soil Association has the most stringent requirements for animal welfare, allowing flocks of no more than 500, which must have free access to organic pasture.

Meat ॐ Organic meat is not only less fatty, it is also free of pesticide residues and growth hormones, plus on organic farms animal welfare is paramount. I was very upset, but not surprised, by the BSE crisis. It demonstrated to me the deep wrongs we are perpetrating on our land and to our livestock.

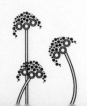

An Organic Life

Pyres are burning

England is a churning

As nature turns to rage

London is burning

As farmers are churning

It's on the front of every page

The world is burning

As nature is churning

With the wrong we do in this age

❦❦❦

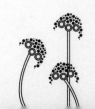

Poultry ✄ Organic chicken, duck and turkey are free range as
well as free of the hormones and antibiotics fed to non-organic
poultry to stimulate growth. You can be sure also that the food
the birds ate will not have been exposed to pesticides.

Fish ✄ Much better for you than animal protein, although is true
that traces of the pesticides that lurk at the bottom of our rivers
and coastal areas have been found in most species. Traces of
mercury are found in most fish too – the larger predators such
as swordfish, shark or marlin have the highest concentrations.
Tuna, especially lightmeat canned tuna, and mackerel have
lower levels. The best route is to eat a variety of fish, as that way
you won't be overexposed to a particular pesticide. Choose wild
fish or organic farmed fish over non-organic farmed fish, which
are doused in organophosphates to kill parasites such as sea-lice
and fed a food colouring to make their flesh the orange colour
it would be in the wild. Non-organic fish farming can also have
a harmful impact on the local ecosystem.

Bread ✄ Organic bread has a higher nutritional value as it contains
more protein, calcium, vitamin A and folic acid. Non-organic
wheat is soaked in chemicals before and after harvesting.

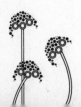

Organic Artisan Bread

I want to say a bit more about bread because I love it! That is, I love bread baked the old-fashioned way, so that it's full of flavour with a denser texture and, of course, packed full of nutrients. There's really no comparison between this artisan-baked bread and the bland factory-produced products that are available in the supermarkets. In the 1960s, our bread production became industrialised and most bread today is made using what is called the Chorleywood Bread Process. This uses low protein wheat, chemical improvers and high-speed mixing and proving, with the result that what you may think of as a natural product contains a surprising list of ingredients. In addition to flour, yeast and water, you may find flour improver, yeast enhancer, fat, a reducing agent, emulsifiers and preservatives. The process also uses chemical enzymes, but they do not have to be listed as they are used up in the bread-making process.

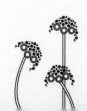

Even organic bread, if it is made by the same large bakery companies, is made by this factory method, though there are stricter rules on the additives that can be used and, of course, the wheat itself is free from chemical residues.

Making bread this way means that much more yeast is needed to get that spongy texture – perhaps this is what lies behind the rise in yeast intolerances and candida?

Artisan or craft bread is made without any artificial additives – basic breads should contain only flour, water, salt and yeast. Sourdough bread may not even contain yeast. The dough is allowed to rise naturally, so that it is full of flavour, with a lovely texture. It's really worth seeking out your local artisan baker – you won't be disappointed.

Jo Fairley, my friend and fellow organic supporter, has a wonderful bakery in Hastings. If ever you are in Hastings, it is well worth popping in.

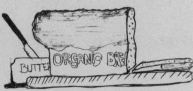

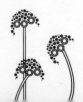

GM FOODS

It's not a new idea to try to breed plants that are stronger with an increased ability to withstand pests, and for generations farmers have been selecting crops based on their own genetic traits. However, 'biotech' scientists have got in on this (lucrative) act and have discovered ways of altering the genes of crops to affect how they grow – the ultimate aim being to grow more crops more cheaply. It is not known what the environmental and health impacts of these new crops may be – testing is still in its infancy – but more and more consumers are anxious about the effects of GM foods, and the likelihood that seeds from GM crops contaminate neighbouring non-GM crops. The Soil Association and other bodies stipulate that food labelled 'organic' should not be genetically modified.

Organic is a way of life for me now, even more so now that I have a young family.

Jesse Wood

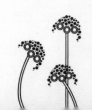

EATING OUT

Going to a fine restaurant is such a pleasure, but it is hard to find organic restaurants, even in London. I am ever hopeful that increasing numbers of restaurateurs will cotton on to the fact that people want organic food, and every time I hear of an organic restaurant opening I make sure I go. It's great to find a wonderful organic restaurant when you least expect it. I was excited to find one called The Wooden Monkey in Halifax in Canada (where the boys were doing a show) and went one evening with Ronnie (of course), and good friends Bernard and Lisa. The food was lovely and the owner, Lil Macpherson, an inspiring woman, who has followed her dream of opening a fantastic organic restaurant.

In non-organic restaurants I always ask if the food is organic. My kids think I'm embarrassing and roll their eyes at each other, but it is too important to worry about niceties. Once I asked a waiter about the food and he insisted, 'Madam, all our food is fresh.' 'Yes, but is it organic?' I asked. 'The chef picks everything himself,' he responded. 'THAT'S NOT THE SAME THING!' I argued the point for ages, trying to make him understand that all I wanted was food that had been grown in natural earth and hadn't been covered in chemicals.

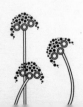

This is important. Please make sure you ask too, and don't worry about what anyone thinks. The more people that make a fuss, the quicker things will change.

KEEP YOUR WITS ABOUT YOU

I go out of my way to get organic everything, even salt and freshly ground black pepper. There is a kind of trick used in supermarkets to get you to buy stuff. Have you noticed all those enticing labels that say 'farm-fresh', 'pure', 'home-grown', 'country style', 'baby new', 'natural wild'? If it doesn't say organic, it's not. And even if it does say organic, check it is properly accredited on the label – look for the logo of a recognizable body like the Soil Association. Don't be fooled!

PESTER POWER

I used to go up to the managers of supermarkets and ask them to stock something organic, or I would ask one of the shelf-stackers to pass a message on. I had read that they like to listen to consumers, so I drove them mad with my requests. Each time I went shopping

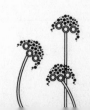

I asked to see the manager of whatever shop I was in. I was always polite, but persistent. 'Why haven't you got any organic food?' I would ask. At first they told me there was no call for it. 'Well, I'm calling for it!' I would respond, and each week I would make the same request. A bit like Jamie Oliver and his school dinners, I was on a one-woman crusade, and I wasn't giving up. When they finally introduced organic cheese in Tesco I was thrilled, but the battle wasn't over. I marched up to the manager (who by now knew me quite well), and declared, 'If you can get me organic cheese you can get me organic butter and organic milk.' And he did. The more I could get, the happier I was.

'You don't really expect celebrities to have any depth to their interest, but Jo has been immensely supportive and genuine. She runs deep, and is a person of great integrity and warmth of heart.'

Patrick Holden, The Soil Association

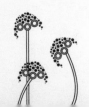

EAT SEASONAL, LOCALLY-PRODUCED FOOD

I know it's really tempting to buy fresh-looking green beans from Kenya in January, enormous Californian strawberries in November, delicious apricots from Chile, sweet mini vegetables from God knows where . . . but don't. Other countries, especially those in the developing world, just don't have the same controls on the use of agricultural chemicals. And not only that, think of the environmental impact of transporting all that stuff halfway across the world, using up fuel and contributing to pollution, just so you and I can have food at the wrong time of year.

We've all got to try to rethink what we cook, when. On the next page is a list of foods that are in season, in this country, each month. Remember when you were little – you didn't expect to have strawberries in winter, did you? Nor did you expect clementines in the summer. We need to get back to the real world and start living in harmony with the seasons. Grow your own, and support your local farmers by going to farm shops, pick-your-own, or farmers markets. They need all the help they can get. If their business does well they will be able to employ more local people, and just by buying direct you reduce the amount of carbon dioxide emissions associated with distribution by 99 per cent. Packaging is reduced, waste is reduced,

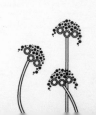

the food is fresher and you'll find a wider range of varieties. At farmers markets, the stallholder is usually the farmer who actually produces the food. If you want to know about the breed of cattle, the crops, the varieties, why they produce what they do, you'll find them happy to chat. Check out *www.farmersmarkets.net* to find your nearest one.

The list on the next page gives a rough guide to what you should particularly look for each month – and what, if you're smart, will be coming up in your garden or allotment. Of course, the months run into each other a little, so it's not a hard-and-fast guide. Several vegetables, such as potatoes, cabbages, onions and carrots, have long seasons.

'It scares me to think how my family and I would be eating now if it wasn't for my sister, who lovingly persuaded me to go organic.'

Lize McCarron, Jo's sister

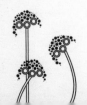

An Organic Life

What's in Season

January ᴆ kale, kohlrabi, leeks, swede, winter radish, winter cabbage, cauliflower, Swiss chard, rosemary

February ᴆ rhubarb (forced), carrots, chicory, Savoy cabbage, parsnips

March ᴆ purple sprouting broccoli, nettles, spring onions

April ᴆ morel mushrooms, new potatoes, spring greens, watercress, outdoor rhubarb

May ᴆ asparagus, broad beans, beetroot, peas, radishes, rocket

June ᴆ broccoli, cucumber, globe artichokes, turnips, peas, samphire, elderflower, soft fruits such as gooseberries, blackcurrants, cherries, raspberries

July ᴆ beans (broad, French and runner), fennel, shallots, cucumber, blueberries, strawberries

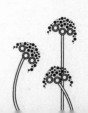

Eating Organically

August ᧐ aubergines, courgettes, squash, sweetcorn, tomatoes, cobnuts, apples, blackberries, plums, pears

September ᧐ mushrooms, swede, kale, blackberries, greengages, damsons, sloes, crabapples, tomatoes

October ᧐ squash and pumpkins, Jerusalem artichokes, Brussels sprouts, red cabbage, celeriac, celery, parsnips, apples, chestnuts, quince

November ᧐ cauliflower, pears, Brussels sprouts

December ᧐ chestnuts, parsnips, red cabbage

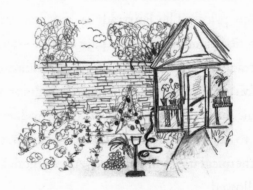

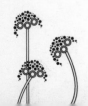

FAIR TRADE

If you're interested in organic food for reasons other than the fact that it tastes better, you will be concerned about the environment and about the conditions in which food is produced. Many producers in the developing world are living in poverty thanks to the unfair nature of global trade – while we reap the benefits in terms of cheaper imported food. And the introduction of monoculture has, in some areas, had a devastating effect on the environment (for instance, the intensive banana production in Costa Rica has seen the forests cut down, the rivers polluted by chemicals and workers suffering from the toxic effects of pesticides). The Fairtrade movement, which began in the 1980s, estimates today that it is helping about 1 million producers and farmers by ensuring they receive fair terms of trade and fair prices. The Fairtrade system also ensures that workers on plantations and factories are paid decent wages and have the right to join trade unions. Child and forced labour are not allowed.

Fairtrade does not mean the products have to be certifiably organic, although it does mean that producers and manufacturers have to follow environmentally sound agricultural practices, and agrochemical use is minimised. Also genetically modified crops are not allowed.

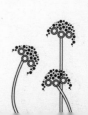

Eating Organically

Once I started learning more about the benefits of an organic lifestyle, I wanted all my friends to know about what was being done to their food. I know that the best way to change people's behaviour is not to hassle them or to make them feel guilty, but to show them the upside. For many years now my family have been holding an annual 'WoodFest' on a summer's evening in the garden of our house in Kingston. The garden always looks magical, with twinkly lights and different themes in different areas – a dance floor in one corner, some of the more talented guests playing in another, chill-out tents, free-flowing champagne – and of course we only serve organic food and drink. Last year we used Planet Organic's wonderful juice people to mix up fantastic juices (see page 213), and alongside the vodka shots guests were offered a single or double shot of bright green wheatgrass juice – an amazing combination! I like to think I've converted a good few people this way.

We always give people something to take home. The year we got back from the Forty Licks tour I was wondering what to put in the goody bags when Craig Sams kindly offered some Green & Black's organic chocolate and Patrick Holden from the Soil Association promised 'something special' from his 240-acre organic farm in Wales. He turned up with 200 bunches of washed, trimmed and neatly tied carrots. A perfect accompaniment to the chocolates!

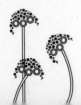

An Organic Life

Last year I celebrated my fiftieth birthday, and I wasn't allowed to have anything to do with the preparations. Everyone was going around the house whispering and giggling and it was driving me crazy not knowing. 'What are we eating?' I kept asking. 'It had better all be organic!' 'Don't worry, Mum, just go and do some yoga and take your mind off it,' they said. The morning of the party dawned, and a big lorry arrived outside. I went to check the food and see if it was organic, as I do, and asked the driver, 'Do you know if this food is all organic?' And he said, 'You bet! It's all come from Jamie Oliver.' Oh, damn! Just spoilt my birthday surprise – but how fantastic! My favourite chef cooking my birthday dinner personally. I was thrilled!

Most of the Stones have come round to my organic way of thinking. Mick is pretty healthy, and Charlie is too, especially after his cancer scare. I got Jerry Hall and Patti into organic, but the one nut I have yet to crack is Keith. He loves an argument, and always takes the mickey out of me for what I'm doing. He's still a wild man at heart – but even wild men have to eat, and I happen to know where Patti does her shopping.

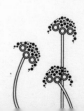

COOKING WITH ORGANIC FOOD

OK, I hope that I've done enough to convince you to become organic from now on. Here are some tips on getting the maximum benefit from what you buy:

🐝 Plan a week's menus in advance, or as soon as you get your organic box delivered (see pages 113–213 for some recipes to get you started). If there is something you're not sure about, make a soup out of it.

❀ As soon as fruit or vegetables are picked, the nutritional content declines, so keep everything in the larder, fridge or a dark cool cupboard. If you're not going to eat or cook it for more than three days, wash, chop and freeze.

🐝 Don't prepare fruit and vegetables hours before you intend to cook them, as they will oxidise and lose loads of the lovely vitamins, minerals and enzymes.

❀ Cook only briefly, with just a small amount of water, or steam, so that you retain the maximum nutritional benefit.

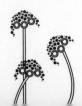

🐝 Save your cooking water for soups and stocks.

🌼 Save energy by cooking double or triple quantities and freezing the extra.

None of the above is new advice, of course. I am arguing for a return to the way our mothers and grandmothers cooked. I remember my granny telling me about making meals out of potato peelings in the war. Nothing was wasted, and everything was fresh. At home we kept chickens, and we had a vegetable patch – even an avocado tree! My earliest memories are of my mother digging up potatoes and making wonderful soups and stews.

'Jo was the first one to tell me about GMOs and going organic. she was just as enthusiastic then as she is now. I love her devotion to organic products. Thanks Josephine, love Patti.'

Patti Hansen Richards

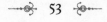

A Healthier, Greener Kitchen

Chop and prepare vegetables on a sheet of newspaper. Gather it all up and chuck it in the compost bin, newspaper and all.

Save water by running full dishwasher loads on the economy cycle.

Try to cut down on packaging and disposables.

Use loose tea instead of teabags.

Shop with canvas or string bags – say goodbye to plastic bags, or at the very least reuse them.

Rather than using kitchen foil or clingfilm, cover bowls with a side plate.

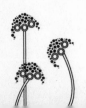

- Use cotton dishcloths, they last longer than sponges; cut up old shirts and sheets for cloths.

- Avoid paper towels and napkins.

- Use pans made from enamelled cast iron, glass or stainless steel. Avoid aluminium and non-stick because of chemical contamination of food.

- Buy non-perishables in bulk, avoiding excess packaging.

'If everyone was as educated as Jo about organic food the world would be healthier and wiser and organic food would be cheaper.'

Vini Karslake, Jo's brother

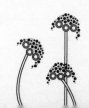

Eating Organically

EDUCATING THE FAMILY

I knew instinctively from the day that I met Gerald that from then on I would not eat another chemical. Like any convert, I was fanatical, and, of course, immediately embarked on educating the whole family. At first I went in pretty hard, and chucked out all the cereals and biscuits they were used to eating, and tried to start them on my radical diet. These were kids who had grown up in America, who had travelled around the world with us eating whatever and whenever. When you're on tour you can't always stop and have a homemade casserole, you grab a takeaway. Not surprisingly, Jamie freaked.

'Where are my Fruity Pebbles?' he demanded. 'Where are my Twinkies?'

'You're sixteen now,' I retorted. 'Time to start eating healthily.'

Nothing would stand in my way. I was curing myself of my illness and I was helping my family too – good health was something I could not ignore. Jamie was going through a difficult stage, I reasoned, he was a little strung out, he was hanging out with a bad crowd (he'd recently got back from a spell in Ibiza). In my mind, I think I imagined a proper diet would get him back on the straight and narrow. I had fond visions of cosy family dinners and delicious

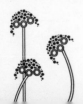

homemade stews. It didn't work, and Jamie steadily became more and more annoyed. One night I discovered he'd sneaked in with a boil-in-the-bag curry.

'You can't eat this!'

'Hey, can't we have any nice-tasting food any more?' he exploded. 'Your food is horrible.'

'It's organic, it's healthy,' I reasoned.

'Well I like my vegetables without worms and manure on them. I like bacon sandwiches with proper white Sunblest bread, it's just not the same all brown and covered in seeds. You've got to stop doing this to me, it's cruel.'

'This wasn't just organic, this was wheatgrass and organic dishwashing powder. Mum took things to the next level: extreme organic.'

Jamie

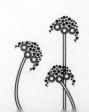

Eating Organically

At last I realised I'd have to be more subtle about the changes I wanted to bring about: as long as it looked like macaroni cheese or spag bol they'd eat it. My challenge was to make them think they were eating the same food, but to use only organic produce and avoid anything processed. I could do pizzas, I could make fish fingers. In fact, Leah, Tyrone and Jesse were fine about the new food; they were young enough to go with whatever I served up. I didn't need to change their diet as wholeheartedly as I was changing mine. And Ronnie was great; he ate whatever I put in front of him and listened to me blathering on about the organic movement for hours on end. He even submitted to organic cigarettes. But it seemed it was too late for Jamie, and the arguments with him continued. He hated what he called the bland, boring tastes:

'Why can't we go to McDonald's any more?' he would grumble.

We were coming from two different planets, I can see that now. I was an evangelist from a new, healthy world and he was just discovering the pleasures of being a teenager – the very pleasures I had spent my life until that point enjoying. I couldn't even tempt him with organic burgers and homemade fried chicken. In the end we decided to leave him to his own devices and he moved out shortly after. On his last evening I cooked him an organic fillet steak. After a few mouthfuls he stopped in surprise.

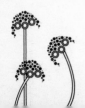

'This is truly the most wonderful thing I have ever tasted, Mum,' he said sadly. 'But I'm still leaving.'

I had to let him go. I realised the time had come for him to stand on his own two feet, so he moved to a small flat in Twickenham. He's always been independent and I admire that tremendously. It is perhaps because of that that we managed to retain a great relationship with each other. I was therefore delighted when, out of the blue, a couple of years later, he called and asked, 'Can I move back home, Mum?'

Today, Jamie works as my manager and, I think, relishes telling me what to do. But that doesn't stop me checking up on him and his eating habits. 'Is it organic?' I have been known to demand, while he groans. I always check his fridge when I am at his house, but I like to think that my perseverance has paid off and he eats a healthy, organic diet. That's what he tells me, anyway.

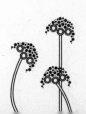

'**I was a very young child when Mum introduced organic everything.** I feel like she's given me a great start in life: organic food is just normal food to me. I feel guilty if I buy anything non-organic but I do sometimes sneak in a quick Chinese takeaway or a Dominos pizza. She always guesses.'

Tyrone Wood

3

Growing Your Own

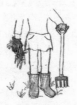

As I've said, I started growing my own vegetables because I couldn't find what I wanted in the shops. I started out of necessity, but it quickly became fun. That sense of being in touch with the earth, of producing my own food for my family from nothing but a handful of seeds was incredibly empowering. I find such joy in feeling in tune with the planet and the seasons, to eat food that I have planted, nurtured, harvested and cooked myself. I have certainly had my disasters, including crops that failed completely, but Patrick, my gardener, and I learnt together. We would hang out together and chat about what we could grow, find some proper organic seeds, and off we'd go. Now I grow all sorts of things in my gardens, from root vegetables, onions and corn, to salads and edible flowers.

WHAT IS ORGANIC GARDENING?

Organic gardening is gardening without manmade pesticides, herbicides or fertilisers. It is gardening that keeps in mind the creation of a healthy, balanced soil, and supports the creatures that find a home in it, such as worms, fungi, bacteria and beetles. In fact, the whole garden benefits from an organic approach, since a healthy soil supports creatures above the ground too, such as birds and insects. The aim is for the insects that eat your plants to be eaten by their natural predators. Thus a healthy soil leads to healthy plants.

The problem with manmade fertilisers is that they do not provide a wide variety of key minerals, vitamins, trace elements, fibre, protein and calories. Organic fertilisers do, and moreover they release the nutrients slowly and naturally. Synthetic fertilisers cause plants to grow quickly, which can make them vulnerable to disease. The other problem with these non-natural chemical fertilisers is the enormous amount of energy used to manufacture them.

You can make your own organic fertiliser by composting – it's easy and fun to do. Just collect your lawn clippings and kitchen waste (such as fruit and vegetable peelings, though avoid meat, eggshells and cooked food as they will attract rats), then ask your council to supply you with a composting bin. It'll come with instructions.

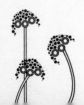

Better still, make your own out of wooden stakes and chicken wire, or wooden pallets. Virtually all gardening manuals will tell you how to do this, or you can check the Garden Organic website for instructions. After a few months (at least three, so you'll need to be patient), when the compost is ready, mulch it around the base of your plants. What you produce may not be certifiably organic according to the Soil Association's rigorous standards, but it will be pretty good. And if you know an organic pig or cattle farm, get hold of some organic manure.

You can grow vegetables almost anywhere, but they'll thrive best in well-drained soil in partially sunny areas of your garden or allotment. I imagine, if it's anything like mine was, your soil is hard and hasn't been cultivated for years – if ever. So, before you start, find out if you've got acid or alkaline soil (your garden centre will sell you a testing kit). If it's alkaline, you'll do well with apples, the cabbage family, sprouts and broccoli, root vegetables, and salad crops. If it's acidic, potatoes, tomatoes and fruit will thrive. Ideally, you'll have neutral soil, in which case you can grow most things.

This is what my gardeners advise:

🐝 Start in the autumn, after a good downpour of rain, but before the first frosts.

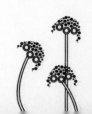

❀ Dig out your soil yourself if you're strong, or use a rotovator if you're not (these are easy to hire), making trenches as you go and filling them with manure or well-rotted compost.

🐝 Use fine potting compost to sow seeds under cloches in March/April, then plant them out in May when the danger of frost has passed.

❀ Don't be discouraged if it takes some time to build up chemical-free soil and if, in the meantime, pests have a go at your crops. Organic gardening is about reducing the effect of pests and diseases on your plants, rather than killing them. Eventually, the pest-eaters will return to your garden, so it's worth persevering.

🐝 Look out for varieties of vegetables that are resistant to fungi or slug attack.

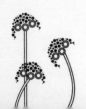

Throw Away the Sprays and Ditch the Pellets

Remember that most insects are to be encouraged because they either eat other insects, or are eaten by larger predators. Get over your instinct to reach for the bug spray, and let the natural world take over. In addition, think about including some of the following in your garden:

- A pond – they are great for attracting a whole host of creatures.

- Piles of logs or leaves will encourage insects and hedgehogs.

- Grow wild flowers in the grass between fruit trees to encourage insects such as hoverflies.

- Honeysuckle is a good place for birds to nest, plus it smells fantastic.

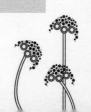

Long grass will attract insects and butterflies.

Encourage birds into your garden by leaving out birdseed or erecting a bird table.

Buddleia and sedum attract butterflies.

Plant holly, berberis and cotoneaster – their berries attract birds.

Keep a nettle patch for butterflies to lay their eggs on, and for you to make nettle soup with.

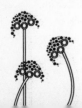

Tips for a Chemical-free Garden

It's much easier to be chemical-free than you think.

- Start a compost heap – this is the single most important thing you can do.

- Prune fruit trees to let in light and air. This goes some way towards avoiding diseases.

- Divide your vegetable plot into beds and make sure there is space for weeding.

- Plant flowers at the end of your vegetable rows to attract predatory insects. I plant Californian poppies and marigolds to attract hoverflies. They look pretty, too.

- Deal with weeds by mulching, hoeing and digging – it's hard work, but think of it as good exercise.

- Cut your grass on a 'short cut' so that clippings left on the lawn fertilise it.

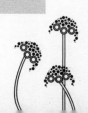

FERTILISERS

I use well-rotted horse manure and my own kitchen compost. To enrich the soil still further, we try other, more unusual techniques, such as growing chives at the base of fruit trees to add nutrients. If we have a glut of something, the leftovers are often dug back into the soil, again as a way of boosting the nutrient content.

CROP ROTATION

This sounds so boring, doesn't it? I'm always reminded of history lessons about the agricultural revolution. But when it came to planting vegetables for our third year, my gardener started going on about it. 'You've got to do crop rotation,' he insisted. 'No,' I said, happy with the way things were. 'I'm sure it will be fine, let's leave the vegetables where they are.' This was before I had learnt about the dangers of monoculture. Patrick agreed to go along with my wishes, no doubt just to teach me a lesson. And, guess what? It wasn't fine at all – the potatoes were awful! Only then did I realise that crops grown in the same place each year take the same nutrients from the soil and therefore weaken the next crop. You need to give the soil

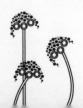

another type of plant to nurture. I also understood why non-crop rotated plants are sprayed with weedkillers – leaving the same crops in the same place year after year allows the diseases to thrive.

Now things are different. We sit and chat about what we're going to plant over a four-year period, and move the different crops around one space as we go. Each month brings fresh excitement in the garden – something to pick, something to plant, something to tend. Every three years it is a good idea to let a bed lie fallow (empty) to give it a rest. Even better, plant some green manure or non-edible beans: when they start to flower just dig them back into the bed.

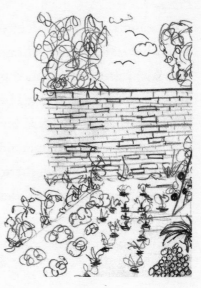

Green manure is a special mix of seeds from plants that naturally release goodness (nitrogen) back into the soil. It comes in three types: field beans for heavy soil, mustard for poor soil and phalecia for all types of soil. Sow from late spring right through to autumn.

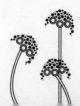

Eating Organically

January

It's so cold outside that seeds need to be sown in pots in the greenhouse. We sow herbs, hardy lettuces and radishes and start sprouting early seed potatoes. My lovely gardeners – Patrick in Ireland and Jeff in London – prepare the ground for new crops, mulching all the beds with my lovely organic compost, which fertilises the plants, enriches the earth and keeps the frost off.

February

This is when it gets really freezing, and I find myself rushing out to grab some chard or carrots then dashing back into the warm house for some hot ginger tea. It's a busy month for digging, sowing and planting, though. On less bitter days I can be found helping to sow early carrots, parsnips and summer cabbages, tucking them up with fleece to protect them against frost. Other seeds that were sown in autumn, such as shallots, broad beans and spinach get planted out now.

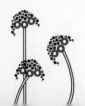

March

What a relief it is when the days start lengthening and you can actually feel the sun on your skin. On warm days, it can be tempting to plant out delicate seedlings too soon, but frosts are still a feature this month. The seeds to sow this month are Brussels sprouts, leeks, peas, broad beans and cauliflower, as well as peppers, courgettes and cucumbers. Chitted potatoes (i.e. ones that have sprouted) should be planted out too, as well as artichokes, onions, garlic and asparagus. Some of the stronger herbs like parsley, chives and feverfew can be moved outdoors.

April

Don't you just love it when the clocks go forward and everyone has a spring in their step? Things get pretty busy in the greenhouse in April and it becomes jam-packed with trays of seedlings for the summer crops. I sow beetroot seeds, sweetcorn, radishes, turnips and carrots, as well as my favourite greens, spinach, kale and Swiss chard, plus loads of herbs. One year we sowed beef tomatoes, which turned out to be enormous; another year our baby yellow plum tomatoes were delicious.

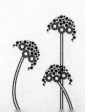

Try yellow courgettes for a change – although remember you're unlikely to need more than three courgette plants as this vegetable really knows how to produce! The first year I grew courgettes we planted 20 and had them coming out of our ears. I like to leave a few courgettes on the plant for a few weeks to allow them to grow into huge marrows.

May

Things start to motor in the garden this month, because of the increased sunlight and late spring showers. We sow autumn vegetables now, such as cabbage, swedes, turnips and squashes. As soon as the danger of frost is past, I plant out some of the summer crops I have been growing from seed over the past few months. Make sure you plant your crops in succession, otherwise you'll have a glut as everything will be ready to harvest at the same time.

June

This is a lovely month, but watering and weeding are a major headache and I try my best to get the kids and their friends to help. I plant out

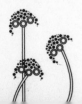

the rest of the summer crops – runner beans, sweetcorn, courgettes, melons – and we carry on sowing winter vegetables, but outside into the beds rather than under cover. Ready to pick this month are the edible flowers – nasturtiums, English marigolds and borage – and soft fruits such as strawberries.

July

Another month to watch weeds, pests and diseases. If you don't harvest your crops in time, they can rot rapidly. I carry on planting lettuces, cabbage, chicory, chard, winter cabbage, peas and carrots. I also pick herbs and dry them on a muslin cloth in the airing cupboard. Leah and I get great pleasure digging everything up together in the summer months.

August

Plants grow like mad in the warm soil, so I carry on planting leeks, cauliflower and cabbage. On the sowing front, I do spring cabbage,

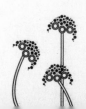

endive, spring onions, fennel and lettuce. In warm weather, to stop crops 'bolting', or going to seed, pinch out the tops.

September

There's loads to pick in September, plus lots of bottling and pickling to do. This month also marks the start of the first cold nights. I sow radishes, spinach, lettuce and cauliflowers outside; and inside I sow early vegetables, herbs and pak choi.

October

I need to watch out for my tender plants in Ireland because autumn seems to set in earlier over there. Many of them get brought inside, and in both gardens I'm out with my cloches to protect peas, winter lettuces and broad beans, and straw to cover celery tops. I plant new potatoes in thick compost. There's bare earth left behind after harvesting and we (or, if I'm honest, Patrick) dig it over thoroughly.

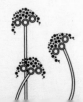

Growing Your Own

November

This is when I bow out and leave the heavy work to the professionals. On damp, foggy days I like to go out and help by raking up leaves to make leaf mould – the soil loves it. I put them in plastic sacks punctured with holes to let the air in.

December

I'm always surprised how much you can still harvest in December – celery, parsnips, swedes, carrots and leeks, as long as the frost doesn't get them first. If you have picked a sheltered spot, or plant against a south-facing wall, some plants will go on for a little bit longer. We can pick parsley virtually all year round, and I harvest miner's lettuce (corn salad, a winter alternative to lettuce), kale and cabbage to add to soups in winter. I know there are some things that can be planted in December, but I'm normally too occupied with parties and preparation for Christmas to do anything terribly active in the garden.

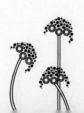

FRUIT

I love an abundance of fresh, homegrown fruit and fortunately we have loads of it. It never goes to waste, as I love baking pies and making jams, chutneys and delicious smoothies (see my suggestions on pages 191–213). We have espalier (fan-trained) fruit trees against our high brick walls, and have managed to grow apricots, peaches, plums, cherries, apples and pears successfully. I also have a fruit cage, which is covered with a net to ward off birds. In it I grow currants, gooseberries, blackberries, raspberries and strawberries. Strawberries can be extra work, but are so worth it! They send out lots of runners with baby plants attached at intervals. These we pot up and grow on for the next year's crop. The other fruits need very little attention, other than pruning out of season and keeping the weeds down.

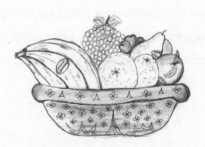

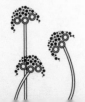

Growing Your Own

VEGETABLES

One of the great things about growing your own vegetables is the huge variety available to you. I love chard and horseradish, which you rarely (if ever) see in supermarkets, mustard greens, which give a great bite to salads, yellow courgettes, which add unusual colour, and tiny new broad beans, which are amazingly tender. It is also possible to grow wonderful fruit varieties, many of which are much tastier than the supermarket alternatives.

I'm lucky to have the space to grow lots of food, but even if you only have a small garden you could try growing strawberries in a pot, or runner beans up a cane wigwam amongst your flowers. In fact, quite a few vegetables can be grown in pots or growbags – tomatoes are particularly easy to grow this way and taste delicious picked when they are fully ripe and warm from the sun. Herbs, too, are a great starting point. You could also try planting aubergines, courgettes or cucumbers in growbags or pots. Not only is it fun, it's also incredibly satisfying to eat food you've grown yourself.

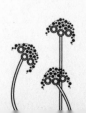

It's a bonding between two

It's a fun thing to do

It puts you in touch with nature

Let's pick another tater

We'll bring it back home and eat it
a bit later

Me and my mum

Leah Wood

4

Food for Health

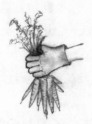

I'VE ALREADY TOLD YOU HOW MY WORLD shifted gear when I met Gerald, the lovely herbalist in Hastings all those years ago. It sparked off an enduring interest in diet and how it affects our health. I read widely and tried out various approaches. The one that seems to make most sense to me – and makes me feel really well and full of energy – is one based on the theory that eating a diet high in alkaline foods is best. The ancient Indian mystics understood this, and the approach underlies Ayurvedic medicine. It is also one of the principles underlying the Hay Diet and food combining. These days, I visit the nutritionist Dr Joshi, either every month or every six months, depending on my needs. Dr Joshi boosts my immune

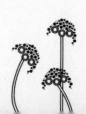

system with acupuncture and gives me whatever supplements I require. If I need it, I'll follow his detox programme. It's not a fast, it's not even a soup-only diet, it's quite unlike most other detox diets you may have come across. It is called 'detox' because a truly alkaline diet will cleanse the system. The strange thing is that his advice is very similar to the original guidelines I was given at Shangri-La.

I keep his detox diet sheet pinned to a noticeboard in my kitchen. I don't stick to it religiously, but I know that when I do follow it I feel at my best. It's important to check with a health care practitioner before detoxing, by the way, just in case you have an undetected medical condition. So when I detox, it's out with booze, red meat (which I rarely eat anyway), dairy, wheat, yeasty and sugary foods, and in with loads of vegetables, pulses, brown rice, probiotic yoghurts and good oils. Good oils include hemp and flax oil, although I'd also like to put in a good word for coconut oil here. Yes, it is a saturated oil, but new research suggests that – unlike other saturated fats such as butter and animal fat – it actually produces energy not fat. Composed of healthy medium-chain fatty acids, coconut oil does not have a negative effect on blood cholesterol, nor does it fur up our arteries. It is safe to heat and cook with, it is a natural antimicrobial (meaning it kills bugs) and is great for improving the quality of skin and hair.

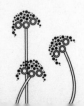

The Alkaline Diet

Our bodies are highly complex mechanisms driven by countless chemical reactions, and balanced body chemistry is crucial for optimum health. We know that acid rain in the environment damages the world around us, but we rarely think about how internal acidity damages our insides. In fact, our modern diet is very high in acid-forming foods, and this results in chronic, low-grade acidosis – or over-acidity in the body tissues. As foods are digested, or 'burned' in the body, they leave a residue behind. This can be neutral, acid or alkaline, depending on the food. A healthy body should be roughly four parts alkaline to one part acid. If it drops to three to one you will be in danger of becoming ill. What happens when we consume too many acid-forming foods is that our bodies go into overdrive to try to neutralise them, interrupting important cellular activities and various bodily functions – including borrowing precious

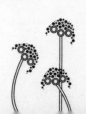

alkalis from our bones. The result? Low energy levels, aches and pains, poor digestion and excess weight, as well as more serious problems such as osteoporosis, diabetes and heart disease. Ideally, about 75 per cent of our diet should be made up of alkaline foods and 25 per cent acidic foods. Almost all fresh fruit, vegetables and pulses are alkaline, while animal products, most grains, processed and junk food are acidic.

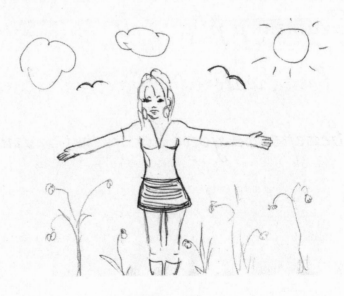

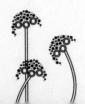

Drinking lots of water is also important. Our bodies are made up of 75 per cent water, and all bodily processes take place in water. If you don't get enough you'll be prone to anxiety, stress, depression, painful joints, painful periods and constricted blood vessels. Drinking 6–8 tall glasses of filtered water each day is essential – it flushes unwanted toxins from your body and keeps your brain sharp. I believe that colas and other fizzy drinks will become the cigarettes of the future.

Examine a plant before and after being watered and relate these benefits to your body and brain.

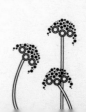

Eating Organically

FOODS TO AVOID

The following is a list of foods you should avoid when on the Alkaline Diet, taken from Dr Joshi's fantastic book, *Dr Joshi's Holistic Detox*:

Alcohol, especially wine, champagne and beer
Yeast and yeast products, such as soy sauce, pickles, Marmite
Bread and other wheat and gluten products
Dairy
Sugar
Chocolates, cakes, biscuits
Tea and coffee, except for herbal varieties
Tomato ketchup, vinegar, mustard
Deadly nightshade family: potatoes, aubergines, cucumbers,
courgettes, tomatoes, peppers
Fizzy drinks
Baked beans
Pizza
Fried and spicy foods
Red meat
Mushrooms
All fruit and juices, except bananas
Nuts, except pine nuts and seeds

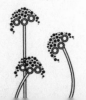

Food for Health

PERMITTED FOODS

The following is a list of foods you can eat when on the Alkaline Diet, again taken from Dr Joshi's book, *Dr Joshi's Holistic Detox*:

Gluten-free oatmeal made with rice milk or water
Eggs, in moderation
Salads and steamed vegetables
Dark green vegetables (not avocados)
White meat
Vegetable juices
Soya and tofu products
Live yoghurt
Buffalo mozzarella, goat's cheese, ricotta, cottage cheese
Wheat-, gluten- and yeast-free breads and cereals
Pulses, lentils and chickpeas
Brown rice
Fish, except shellfish, tuna and swordfish
Vegetable soups
Soya, rice and goat's milk
Olive oil

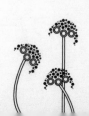

Eating Organically

When I'm not on a rigid detox I still err on the alkaline side: low-carb, with plenty of vegetables and beans and not too much meat, fish and eggs. I avoid junk food and refined carbohydrates. I really miss sugar and chocolate, but organic halva is my treat – it's made of sesame seed and honey, and I think really, how bad can that be?

I love to cook a good steak or lamb chop, but do rarely eat red meat. There are many good reasons to eat more vegetables, an approach that is becoming known as 'eating low on the food chain'.

🌸 More than half the world's grain harvest is used to feed animals reared for their meat.

🌸 Vegetarians have lower rates of heart disease and cancer, are often slimmer than meat eaters, and have lower cholesterol and blood pressure levels.

🌸 Too much protein is harmful, has been linked to degenerative diseases and premature ageing.

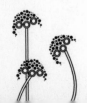

Food for Health

SUPERFOODS

There has been quite a bit in the press about so-called superfoods, and there seems to be considerable disagreement over which ones are the best for you. My motto is, 'If it's colourful, it's good for you', because the dark green, blue, red, orange and yellow foods have so many special, healthy qualities. This is not an exhaustive list, but it's a list of my favourite superfoods. They all pack a punch, and – what's more – are also thought to fight the effects of age. Definitely tastier than botox.

Barley ✧ protects against colon and breast cancer, lowers
cholesterol, contains the 'super' form of vitamin E and the
heart-protecting vitamin B. Whole pot barley contains higher
levels of nutrients than pearl barley, which has had the husk
removed.

Beans and lentils ✧ Full of fibre, antioxidants, folic acid and
potassium, they are a good source of B vitamins and protein
and are low in fat and calories. They are also good for the skin
as the body uses them to produce hyaluronic acid, which we
need to keep the moisture in and the wrinkles away.

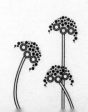

Blueberries ❧ These tiny berries are packed with an astonishing amount of good stuff, including vitamin C, folic acid, fibre and carotenoids, which protect our skin from sun damage, slow down ageing and boost the immune system.

Broccoli ❧ Great for cancer prevention (like all members of the cabbage family), as well as being a good source of vitamin C, beta carotene, iron and folic acid.

Buckwheat ❧ Second to none in lowering cholesterol levels, it is rich in zinc, copper and manganese. It's good for your heart and circulation, and can even reduce high blood pressure.

Oats ❧ Cholesterol lowering, these contain high levels of vitamin B and fibre to keep your gut healthy and your blood sugar low.

Onions, garlic and leeks ❧ These all belong to the 'allium' family and help eliminate toxins, beat cancer, stabilise blood sugar and guard against stomach problems.

Oranges ❧ One of the best ways of getting your vital dose of Vitamin C.

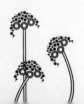

Pumpkin ✺ A good source of betacarotene and vitamin C, and
helps regulate cholesterol levels.

Quinoa ✺ This looks like a grain but is really a seed. It is an
unusually complete protein as it contains the amino acid lysine.
It is high in fibre, iron, potassium and B vitamins as well as
containing magnesium, zinc, manganese, copper, folic acid and
vitamin E. It is gluten free which makes it easier to digest.

Salmon (wild or organic) ✺ The omega 3 fatty acids are great
for your heart and your skin, and it is also a good source of
selenium, copper and zinc.

Soy ✺ Not soy sauce, but products such as tofu, soya milk or soya
nuts. It's a great vegetarian protein – although, as tofu is made
by fermentation with yeast, if your immunity is compromised I
think you'd be best to avoid it.

Spinach ✺ Contains iron, folic acid and vitamin K, which helps
maintain bone health, plus it has anti-inflammatory nutrients.

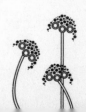

Sprouts ᴚ Not Brussels, but what you get when seeds start to sprout, i.e. alfalfa, broccoli, mung bean, chickpea, lentil or fennel sprouts. These little things are powerhouses of nutrients and enzymes – you can buy them ready-sprouted in health shops, alternatively, try growing them yourself.

Tea (green or black) ᴚ A source of antioxidants, though the highest levels are found in green tea rather than black.

Tomatoes ᴚ A good source of vitamins A, C and E, they also contain the antioxidant lycopene, which reduces the risk of some cancers, especially prostate.

Turkey ᴚ A good source of protein, low in fat and high in energy. Also contains typrophan, which the body uses to produce serotonin, a hormone that boosts our mood and helps us to sleep.

Walnuts ᴚ Contain vitamin E, zinc and omega 3 fatty acid, which lowers cholesterol and decreases your chances of getting heart disease.

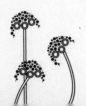

Yoghurt ✦ A rich source of calcium, which helps build strong bones and teeth. Also contains healthy bacteria that aid digestion and are thought to guard against polyps in the gut.

Tea

I want to share with you my obsession with tea, proper tea – not the fruity kind, although I occasionally have a herbal brew. I drink tea all the time, and love sampling new varieties. I like to sit in my drawing room and relax quietly with a cup of oolong tea in the afternoon, savouring the taste, sipping slowly. The most health-giving varieties are green tea and oolong tea.

All teas come from the same plant, *camellia senensis*. What distinguishes the different types from each other is how and where they are grown, and what is done to the leaves once they are picked.

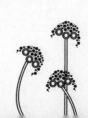

Green tea is the most delicate in flavour. When the leaves are picked they are heated very quickly to prevent the enzymes from oxidising. The ancient Taoists called it 'the elixir of immortality' and certainly it has some amazing properties. It contains polyphenols, free-radical scavengers that prevent cellular deterioration, which in some studies have been shown to protect against cancer. Polyphenols also lower the body's cholesterol and blood glucose levels and help fight asthma and respiratory infections. Green tea also has antibacterial properties, is a natural source of manganese, and contains vitamin P, which strengthens blood vessels. So you can see why it was thought to bestow immortality! To make it, add to water that is not quite boiling.

The name oolong in Chinese means 'black dragon'. It has a more fragrant and aromatic flavour, floral and woody. It is semi-oxidised and therefore is higher in caffeine than green tea. It is good for the heart, helps the body eliminate toxins and lowers cholesterol levels. In addition, it strengthens the

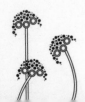

immune system, raises the spirits and stimulates clear thinking. It is also high in vitamins A, B2, D, P and manganese. As with green tea, brew with water that is not quite boiling.

Black tea is the darkest tea and strongest in flavour. The leaves are completely oxidised – which is achieved by a process of heating the leaves in a moist environment. All black teas contain caffeine, but the more oxidised they are, the more caffeine they contain, and the fewer vitamins and polyphenols. Green tea is six times more powerful an antioxidant than black tea. There are various types, but Darjeeling is one of the most popular. Loose tea is best, because tea bags contain the dust or leftovers that are swept out of the tea machines, with the result that the flavour is less subtle and stronger than loose leaf tea.

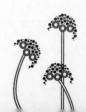

NUTRITIONAL HEALING

You can't have failed to notice the prominence given in newspapers and magazines to the role good nutrition has to play in combating certain illnesses. By now you'll have realised that I'm a complete convert to this way of thinking – I believe that everything from arthritis to varicose veins can be tackled in part by the right foods or herbs. In fact, I'm convinced I wouldn't be here today if I hadn't been put on the correct nutritional path by my friend Gerald. Today, I possess three copies of an enormous bible on nutrition that I use all the time. I take one on tour with me, I have another at home in Kingston and another in Ireland. Whenever I feel ill, which is very rare these days, or a family member is suffering from something or other, I look up the illness and do everything it tells me to do.

Vitamins are organic substances necessary for health. By vitamins I don't necessarily mean pills, although I take my vitamin tablets religiously – not just the special supplements prepared for me by Dr Joshi, but other ones imported from the US. I came across the latter through Ed and Fred, identical twins who make leather straps for guitars. They're hilarious – one starts a sentence, the other finishes it. On a recent tour they gave me some samples of the organic vitamins they were taking. I loved them so much that I ordered a whole load.

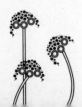

Food for Health

*It's important to take a good multivitamin
and mineral supplement every day.
You never know which small nutrient is the one
your body needs right now.*

A Quick Guide to Vitamins

The best way of taking vitamins is to get them directly from fresh, organic food. Here's a quick guide to the basic ones.

Vitamin A ~ Helps protect against infection, maintains mucous membranes and skin and cell membranes. Good for eye problems, acne, it promotes strong bones and healthy skin, hair and teeth. Sources include apricots, broccoli, carrots, eggs, fish-liver oils, spinach, watercress and watermelon.

Vitamin B1 (thiamin) ~ Essential during illness, stress or surgery. Good for the nervous system, it aids digestion and keeps the muscles and heart functioning well. Sources include bran, egg

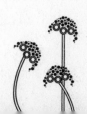

yolks, grains, organic meats, milk, most vegetables, peanuts and fish.

Vitamin B6 ♂ A deficiency can cause exhaustion and anaemia. It is often prescribed for premenstrual tension (PMS), bloating and morning sickness. Sources include brewer's yeast, liver, eggs, oats, walnuts, fish, pulses and vegetables.

Vitamin B12 ♂ Required for red blood cell production and the health of the nervous system. It's good for improving concentration and can relieve irritability. Deficiency can lead to fatigue and anaemia. Sources include eggs, fish, milk and meat.

Vitamin C ♂ Necessary for healthy immune system functioning. A deficiency can be caused by alcohol, cigarettes and stress, which in turn can lead to fatigue, a lowered immune system, colds and flu and arthritis. Sources include fresh fruit and vegetables, particularly bright orange, dark green and red varieties.

Vitamin D ♂ Required for strong healthy bones and for the efficient release of hormones. Sources include cod liver oil,

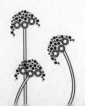

egg yolks, mackerel and sardines. Our bodies use sunlight, converting it to the vitamin.

Vitamin E ↝ Needed for wound healing, healthy muscles and nerves, and for the manufacture of cell walls. Sources include Brussels sprouts, eggs, grains, spinach, pecans and walnuts.

MINERALS

Minerals are also vital to health, albeit in small quantities. We need them to help our bodies absorb the vitamins.

Calcium ↝ Required for healthy bones and teeth, as well as for moderating cholesterol levels. It also aids nerve, muscle and digestive function. Sources include whole grains, pulses, green leafy vegetables, oranges and milk.

Copper ↝ Metabolises the iron in the body and helps prevent water retention. Also needed for healthy skin and hair. Sources include whole grains, mushrooms, olives, pulses, dried fruit, liver, shellfish and nuts.

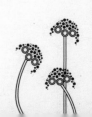

Iron ↷ Carries oxygen around the body and boosts the immune system. Sources include red meat, whole grains, egg yolk, nuts, soya, dark green vegetables, dried fruit and mushrooms.

Potassium ↷ Needed for energy. Also regulates the heart rhythm, transports oxygen to the brain and helps digestion. Sources include whole grains, nuts and seeds, bananas, cabbage, celery, broccoli and peas.

Selenium ↷ Protects the cells against free radicals, regulates the hormones and is needed for a healthy liver, eyes, hair, nails and skin. Sources include nuts (especially brazil nuts), white fish, liver, kidney, cereals, bread and dairy products.

Silica ↷ Helps regenerate skin and keep the wrinkles at bay. Also needed for shiny hair and strong nails, teeth and bones. Sources include whole grains and cereals, onions, soya, root vegetables, beetroot, spinach and leeks.

Zinc ↷ Essential for healthy skin, healing wounds and a healthy immune and reproductive system. Sources include seafood,

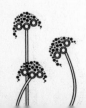

nuts and seeds, beef, sardines, pulses, whole grain cereals, brown rice and green vegetables.

ANTIOXIDANTS

An umbrella term for a bunch of enzymes, vitamins, minerals, supplements and amino acids that protect us from free radicals – uncontrolled oxidants that damage the cells of our bodies, weaken our immune system and lead to diseases such as heart disease and cancer. You will have heard of some of them, vitamins A, C and E for example, but they also include coenzyme Q10, betacarotene, selenium, superoxide dismutase and zinc. As we age, we find it harder to manufacture these ourselves, so it is important to eat foods rich in these antioxidants. In general, the brightly coloured foods do this job best, as well as garlic, onions and leeks, and the cabbage family. Dark chocolate and red wine also, thankfully, contain antioxidants.

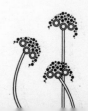

Supplements

Ideally, we would derive all our vitamins and minerals from our food. The nutritional content of much of what we eat, though, is compromised by modern farming practices, and as soon as a piece of fruit is picked or a vegetable is dug up from the ground it starts to lose its vitamins. In addition, many nutrients are destroyed by cooking, and reheating puts paid to the few that remain, particularly if the food is microwaved. Processed foods are virtually devoid of nutrients, yet when we are busy this is often what we eat. For lunch, many of us just grab a sandwich and a cup of coffee and expect it to keep our bodies going all day. These are the reasons we need supplements. As I'm sure you are aware, there are hundreds of supplements available, and it would be impossible in a book like this to list them all. I can do no better than to recommend you to Earl Mindell's *Vitamin Bible*, which is a fantastic guide to what you might need and how to go about getting it.

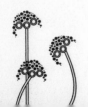

Food for Health

Kitchen Pharmacy

Since learning all about living naturally I have become a bit of a kitchen pharmacist. Whenever a friend or a family member is suffering from something I instantly open my store cupboard, tea chest or box of aromatherapy oils. Stomach upset? I make a slippery elm porridge. Sounds horrible, but it works. Sunburn? Aloe vera straight from the plant, a warm camomile bath, plenty of fluids for rehydration and high-protein foods for tissue repair. Athlete's foot? Avoid sugar and rub garlic and honey into the affected area. For wasp and bee stings, rub lavender oil directly on to the skin. Lavender oil is also an effective insect repellant. Once I got arthritis in my neck and followed the advice in my nutritional bible to the letter. Afterwards, when I went back to my physio, he uttered those memorable words, 'You don't need to come back again.' For arthritis and aches and pains, my mum swears by feverfew which we grow in our garden – it's easy to grab a bunch and bind it to the painful part with a bandage.

The message I want to convey here is: *don't necessarily rush to the doctor for everything* – find out what you can do to help yourself, and get some natural remedies from your health food shop or online. It is incredibly empowering.

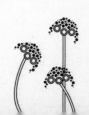

My Mum's Home Remedies
for Common Ailments

AILMENT	AVAILABLE FROM HEALTH SHOP	MAKE UP YOURSELF
ACHES AND PAINS	*arnica cream or tablets* *Tiger Balm™ rub*	*compress of lavender,* *rosemary and majoram* *ice pack, eat food rich in* *vitamin C and zinc*
BITES AND STINGS	*take zinc, thiamine or* *garlic supplements* *to repel insects –* *they hate the smell*	*bees: bicarbonate of soda* *wasps: vinegar or* *lemon juice* *mosquitos: tea tree oil,* *aloe vera* *nettles: dock leaves,* *lavender oil*
BLISTERS	*witch hazel, lavender oil* *aloe vera, calendula cream* *Rescue Remedy™*	*salt water*

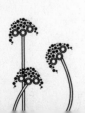

Food for Health

AILMENT	AVAILABLE FROM HEALTH SHOP	MAKE UP YOURSELF
BRUISES	arnica, witch hazel	cold pack, vinegar compress, hot cabbage leaves
BURNS AND SCALDS	aloe vera, lavender oil calendula and hypericum tincture (diluted) for at least 15 mins	hold under cold water apply a cold, wet tea bag
COLDS	mullein tea steam with tea tree, eucalyptus and olbas oil	lemon and honey eat foods rich in zinc and vitamin C drink ginger root and honey tea
CUTS AND SORES	calendula and hypericum cream lavender oil, tea tree oil (diluted) aloe vera gel	salt water, honey
EARACHE	2 drops mullein or St John's Wort oil dripped into the ear	warm olive oil dripped into the ear

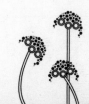

AILMENT	AVAILABLE FROM HEALTH SHOP	MAKE UP YOURSELF
EARACHE (CONT.)	*massage lavender or camomile oil around the ear*	*lie on a water bottle filled with hot, but not boiling water*
GENERAL TONIC OR 'PICK ME UP'		*fresh lemon balm and honey*
HEADACHES	*massage peppermint and lavender oils into temples*	*make tea infusions of one or more of the following herbs: feverfew, meadowsweet, valerian, vervain, ginger root*
HEADLICE	*mix up oils of citronella, lavender, eucalyptus, geranium, rosemary in a carrier oil and comb through hair regularly with a nit comb*	
INDIGESTION		*fennel, peppermint, lemon balm or camomile tea*

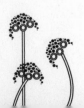

Food for Health

AILMENT	AVAILABLE FROM HEALTH SHOP	MAKE UP YOURSELF
INSOMNIA	lavender oil on pillow or in bath	warm bath camomile, valerian, vervain or lemon balm tea
MOUTH ULCERS	myrrh oil or tincture aloe vera geranium oil mouthwash of lavender oil diluted in water	chew ginger root eat foods rich in B vitamins
NAUSEA	ginger capsules	peppermint tea
SHOCKS	Rescue Remedy™ arnica tablets and cream lavender oil rub	camomile tea
SORE THROAT	thyme oil inhalation gargle with sage tea or tea tree oil	gargle with warm salt water or apple vinegar and honey

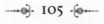

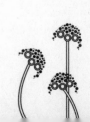

Eating Organically

AILMENT	AVAILABLE FROM HEALTH SHOP	MAKE UP YOURSELF
SORE THROAT (CONT.)	*Massage neck area with lavender oil*	
SUNBURN	*aloe vera, lavender oil*	*cold tea applied to skin drink copious amounts of water*
TOOTHACHE	*apply clove or peppermint oil to tooth*	*garlic clove on tooth, chew sage leaves or garlic*
VERRUCAS AND WARTS	*tea tree oil*	*garlic, lemon juice, or – bizarrely – a banana skin stuck to the offending part of the body with plaster*

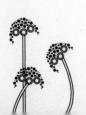

5

Cooking On and Off the Road

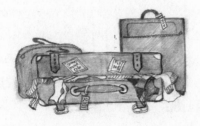

I DIDN'T EXPECT THAT WE'D STILL BE TOURING at this point in our lives. I thought Forty Licks in 2002–2003 would be the last Stones tour, but then A Bigger Bang happened in 2005, and we were off again. I look back over the years and I laugh at how little has changed. The girls are there, all the same loyal fans screaming and most of the people we work with are the same. But, let's face it, we are all that much older and the parties aren't quite so wild. They used to call our room Party Central, but now things are much quieter. Now there is a personal trainer and organic food backstage.

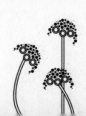

We have quiet dinners out, hook up with friends from all over the world, or just watch a movie.

It's my job to look after Ronnie. About sixteen years ago, Mick came to me and said, 'Ronnie needs an assistant. You're here all the time, so you've got the job.'

'What, you're going to pay me for looking after my husband? Great!'

So I get his wardrobe together, plan every outfit, every change, make sure he is on time and knows what he is doing. I used to do his make up, but now I work with the stylist, William, Isobel, the wardrobe girl, and Caroline, the make-up artist. In fact, we have all worked together on tour for so many years, it is like a family. And now I have my products I am able to promote them while on tour.

Before we leave home I pack a dozen suitcases, each basically representing a drawer of certain clothes – shirts in one, suits in another. I try to be organised and not leave anything to chance. At home I have one whole room devoted to clothes – everything has its place. I let Ronnie choose what he's going to wear on stage, though I pull out a selection of jackets that I know won't clash with what the rest of the guys on stage are wearing, especially Mick, and a choice of T-shirts with colours that will work – that way it makes him feel that the final choice is his.

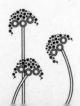

Cooking On and Off the Road

I take care of what Ronnie and I eat on tour. He's always busy, either rehearsing, playing or doing press, so he hasn't got much time to think about food. The first tour after my conversion to all things organic was hard, and I had a dreadful time trying to find organic restaurants and shops, although some cities in the US were pretty clued-up. Eventually I realised that I was going to have to cook my own food, which was fine because I love cooking, but I needed a stove. So I went out and bought a little two-ringed electric burner from a camping shop. It was great – I was suddenly able to cook up organic food in our hotel room and the constant concern over what we were going to eat next evaporated overnight. I stored the stove, wrapped in hotel towels, in a hard suitcase, along with mustard, salt, pepper, tomato sauce, olive oil – all organic, of course – although I was always worried about putting it in the case when it was slightly warm and knew it would be better if I could find another solution.

As always, it was my son Jamie who came to the rescue. At the time, he ran a backstage furniture company and he knows guys who can design pretty much anything. So when we were next back home I sat down with a guy who makes flight cases. He said he could make me a travelling cooker: fab!

'I need a cooker that won't burn the suitcase. I want drawers for food and utensils. I also need to be able to wheel it around and

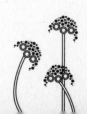

it must close properly.' He nodded professionally, as if I was asking for the most normal thing in the world, and started sketching designs on a piece of paper. In the end he produced the most fabulous creation. Just what I wanted – and more. A hip-height black flight case with two doors that open out into an instant cooker. It boasts two halogen burners that cool down the minute you turn them off, a toaster, kettle, dual voltage, large drawers to store dry food and jars, knives and wooden spoons. It folds up into a neat flight case that looks just like a music system of some kind. I take it everywhere with me now and no concierge has ever raised an eyebrow.

I take a certain amount of food with me, tucked away in the drawers. Organic baked beans, pasta, olive oil, ketchup, mustard powder, spices and dried herbs – anything I don't need to buy fresh. The moment we arrive in a new city and get to our hotel, instead of waiting for our luggage I make a beeline for the nearest health food store, buying up quantities of fresh organic food. Most big cities are fine, and even smaller ones are getting better. But even if we are in some remote town, I know we'll be able to survive on beans. Admittedly, I have sometimes set the smoke alarms off when making toast, but I just fling open the windows and wave my arms madly at the fire alarm and it seems to do the trick.

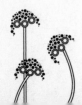

Cooking On and Off the Road

When it comes to cooking on the road on my lovely two-burner stove, meals have to be simple – but I make sure they are tasty, wholesome and nutritious by buying the very best ingredients. Once you have good, organic produce the rest is easy. I love to cook, and love it when our big kitchen at home is full of the sweet smells of cooking and my family is asking me, 'What's for dinner?' I never know quite who is going to turn up to dinner – Leah and her boyfriend Jack, Ty and Nat, my son Jamie and his family or one of a number of musicians or friends. They know that there will always be a big pot of something delicious in the oven. I believe in food as nourishment, rather than something that fills you up when you're in a rush. I think it should be savoured and used as a focal point for talking over the day's events, for regrouping as a family and for making plans and celebrating achievements.

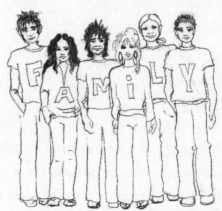

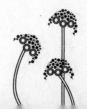

Eating Organically

GOOD COOKING IS ABOUT RESPECT
FOR THE RAW MATERIALS

I have never been one to follow instructions slavishly in cookery books, and most of the time I make things up as I go along, taking a bit from one recipe and adding it to another, going intuitively by taste and eye. I suppose you could say I'm a natural organic cook – as long as my ingredients are organic or straight out of the garden I know I can make a fab meal that's full of nutrition. So, some of the following recipes I have made up, some are adapted from other people's, and some have been handed down to me by my mother and grandmother, or from Ronnie's family. As we live a nomadic life, some are suitable for cooking in a proper kitchen, others are perfect for when we're touring. When we're on the road it's important to have a good breakfast, especially if it has been a long night. So, despite the limitations of my double burner, I'll do bacon and eggs, or scrambled or poached eggs on toast. For dinner I might make fried fish and rice, or garlic prawns and rice, chops and potatoes, steak or sausages and mash. Any of these can be served with a mixed salad – so who says you can't eat healthily on the road? I have tried very hard to make the measurements clear, but I usually rely on handfuls of this or that – so do make adjustments if you wish. Unless otherwise stated, all recipes serve four. And, of course, all ingredients are organic.

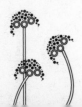

Recipes

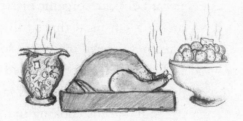

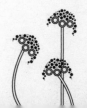

'**All my mates love Mum's cooking** – they secretly love that it's organic but don't admit it.'

Tyrone Wood

Soups

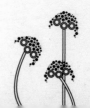

Lentil and Lovage Soup

This is a wonderful, nutritious soup.
I grow lovage in my garden and make this when it's in season.

1 small onion, finely chopped

2 tablespoons extra virgin olive oil

250 g small lentils, rinsed

1 litre hot vegetable stock

2 whole garlic cloves, unpeeled

250 g lovage, cleaned, washed and chopped

2 tomatoes, peeled, deseeded and diced

salt and freshly ground black pepper

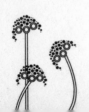

Sweat the onion in the oil in a heavy-
bottomed soup pot until transparent.
Add the lentils and stir for 5 minutes.
Add the boiling stock, along with the garlic,
cover, and simmer for 20 minutes. Add the
lovage, tomatoes and salt. Replace the lid
and simmer for a further 30 minutes until
the lentils are soft, then remove the garlic
and add some freshly ground pepper.
To serve, place a slice of toasted bread in
each bowl and cover with soup.

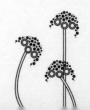

Bean and Coriander Soup

2 tablespoons oil

1 large onion, chopped

1 head of fennel, chopped

2 level teaspoons ground coriander

1.5 litres chicken stock

1 × 400-g can chopped tomatoes

2 level teaspoons tomato purée

1 garlic clove, crushed

bunch of fresh coriander, leaves chopped

and stalks tied together

salt and freshly ground black pepper

1 × 400-g can cannelini beans, drained and rinsed

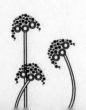

Heat the oil in a large saucepan.
Add the onion and fennel and fry until
just starting to brown. Stir in the ground
coriander and cook for a minute. Add the
stock, chopped tomatoes, tomato purée,
garlic and coriander stalks. Season, bring
to the boil and simmer, covered, for 30
minutes. Just before serving, add the beans
and heat through. Garnish with the chopped
coriander leaves.

*This is a lovely warming soup,
just right for a cold spring day.*

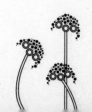

Chickpea and Chard Soup

200 g dried chickpeas

2 garlic cloves

3 fresh sage leaves

30 g dried mushrooms

2 tablespoons extra virgin olive oil

1 celery stick, chopped

1 carrot, chopped

1 onion, chopped

2 tablespoons tomato purée

400–500 g Swiss chard, chopped

salt and freshly ground black pepper

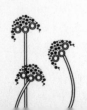

Soak the chickpeas in cold water overnight. Drain, rinse and place in large pot. Add one unpeeled garlic clove, the sage leaves and enough water to cover them with 2 cm to spare. Bring to the boil, cover, and simmer for 2 hours or until the chickpeas are soft and almost completely cooked. Add salt in the last 10 minutes of cooking. Set aside.

Meanwhile, soak the dried mushrooms in hot water for 10 minutes. Strain, squeeze dry and chop. Heat the oil in a large pan and add the celery, carrot, onion, remaining garlic clove, chopped, and the mushrooms. When the vegetables are soft, add the tomato purée. Cook for 5 minutes, then add the Swiss chard. Season with salt and freshly ground black pepper and simmer, covered, until tender. Add the mixture to the cooked chickpeas, and simmer, again covered, for a further 20 minutes. Remove the garlic cloves and sage before serving.

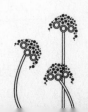

Mushroom Soup

40 g butter

250 g mushrooms (chestnut mushrooms work well)
wiped and finely chopped

25 g plain flour

600 ml hot chicken stock

300 ml milk

1 tablespoon chopped parsley

salt and freshly ground black pepper

1 tablespoon lemon juice

2 tablespoons double cream (optional)

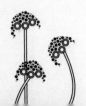

Melt the butter in a large saucepan,
add the mushrooms and cook over a
medium heat for about 10 minutes until
soft. Stir in the flour and cook for a further
minute. Pour in the hot stock and milk and
bring to the boil, stirring constantly. Cover
and simmer for about 10 minutes. Remove
from the heat and, stirring well, add the
parsley, lemon juice and cream, if using.
Adjust the seasoning, then return the pan
to the stove and reheat gently, taking care
not to boil. Pour into warmed soup
bowls and serve.

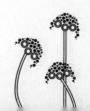

Pumpkin Soup

This lovely autumnal soup can also be made with butternut squash.

1 medium onion, chopped

40 g butter or 2 tablespoons coconut oil

500 g cooked, mashed pumpkin

(about 1 medium pumpkin)

1 teaspoon salt

1 tablespoon sugar

¼ teaspoon nutmeg

¼ teaspoon ground pepper

750 ml hot chicken stock

125 ml cream

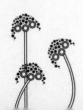

Gently brown the onion in the butter or
coconut oil. Add the mashed pumpkin,
together with the salt, sugar, nutmeg and
pepper. Slowly add the chicken stock and
heat thoroughly, but do not allow to boil.
Pour into a tureen and add the cream.

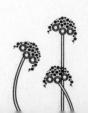

Minestrone

This recipe was given to me by my sister Lize

SERVES 4–6

1 large aubergine, cubed

1 medium onion, chopped

3 garlic cloves, chopped

1 tablespoon olive oil

2 × 400-g cans chopped tomatoes

4 medium carrots, sliced

2 bay leaves

½ glass red wine

1 teaspoon oregano

160 g Penne pasta

240 ml water

salt and freshly ground pepper

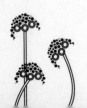

Fry the aubergine, onion and garlic in the
oil in a large, heavy-bottomed pan until
nicely browned. Add the tomatoes, carrots,
bay leaves, wine, oregano and salt and
pepper to taste, and cook, uncovered,
on a medium heat for 20 minutes.
Add the pasta, plus the water, and cook
until the pasta is al dente.
Serve with organic crusty bread.

*This is my favourite recipe for minestrone —
it's a meal rather than a soup.*

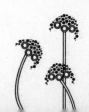

Salads

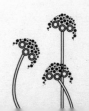

Aduki Bean Salad

250 g aduki beans, soaked overnight in cold water
1 stock cube
2 carrots, diced
1 medium butternut squash, peeled, deseeded and diced
1 medium onion, chopped
1 × 400-g can butter beans

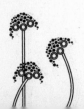

Drain and rinse the aduki beans, place in a large saucepan, cover with cold water, add the stock cube and bring to the boil. Cover with a lid and simmer for 15 minutes, then add the squash, carrots and onion. Cook for a further 15 minutes or until the vegetables are tender. Add the butter beans towards the end of the cooking time and heat through. Drain off any excess cooking liquid and allow to cool slightly before mixing the salad with your own dressing. Serve warm or at room temperature.

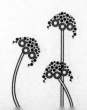

My Energy Salad

4 handfuls (100 g) rocket leaves

6 tomatoes, sliced

2 celery sticks, chopped

2 carrots, grated

12 radishes, halved

2 tablespoons pumpkin seeds

2 cooked beetroots, diced

¼ cucumber, diced

extra virgin olive oil

lemon juice

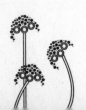

Toss together all the ingredients,
and season with salt and freshly ground
black pepper. Drizzle with extra virgin
olive oil and a squeeze of lemon.

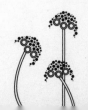

Fish

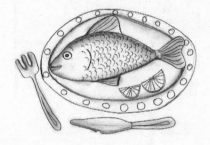

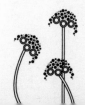

Jo's Famous Paella

*I first had paella on tour in Spain,
and now I always cook it in summer.
It's so easy, plus this is a very forgiving recipe –
I tend to chuck in whatever I have.
Leah and I particularly love it.*

SERVES 6

8 big prawns
1.5 litres bouillon stock
pinch of saffron
1 ½ teaspoons salt
1 tablespoon coconut or olive oil
175 g chorizo sausage, cut into 5-mm slices
4 boneless chicken thighs, cut in half

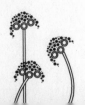

1 medium onion, roughly chopped
1 medium red chilli, deseeded and chopped
2 garlic cloves, chopped
500 g Spanish paella rice
pinch of paprika
1 glass organic white wine
500 g mixed fish, such as cod, salmon,
scallops, whiting, cut into chunks
4 large tomatoes, peeled, deseeded and diced
5 tablespoons chopped parsley
100 g frozen peas
grated zest of 1 lemon

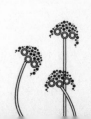

First prepare the stock. Peel the prawns and place the shells and heads in a large pan with the bouillon, garlic, saffron and a pinch of salt. Bring to the boil, then reduce the heat and simmer for 15 minutes. Strain the stock into a jug and then set aside.

Heat the oil in a large pan, add the diced chorizo and chicken thighs. Sauté quickly over a high heat until golden brown, then remove and set aside. Add the onion, chilli and garlic to the pan and fry until the onion is soft and transparent. Stir in the rice and add the paprika. Stir for 2 minutes, then start slowly adding the hot stock and white wine, stirring all the while. It should start smelling delicious. Leave on a low to medium heat for 15 minutes, stirring occasionally.

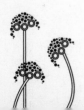

Fold in the chorizo and chicken pieces,
cover, and leave to cook until the rice is
tender and the chicken is cooked through.
Add the mixed fish pieces, chopped
tomatoes, parsley, peas and lemon zest.
Replace the lid and cook for a further
couple of minutes to cook through,
then serve with good red wine.

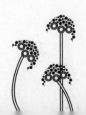

Baked Smoked Haddock

This is nice and easy, and is delicious served with new potatoes and peas. Ronnie and Ty love it, cooked just like Ronnie's mum made it . . . Avoid that orange-tinged haddock you see in supermarkets — it's artificially dyed. Natural smoked haddock, without chemicals or colourings, has a pale golden sheen and a beautifully balanced flavour.

4 fillets undyed smoked haddock
300 ml milk (I use goat's milk)
splash or two of water
knob of butter
black pepper

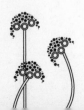

Preheat the oven to 180°C.
Wash the fish and cut each fillet into two
large pieces. Arrange in a shallow ovenproof
dish. Add the milk and water, put a little
butter on each piece of fish and grind some
pepper over the top. Bake in the oven for
20 minutes or until the fish is cooked.
Do not overcook!

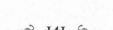

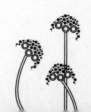

Sea Bass in Organic Salt

Mmm, fabulous. This always reminds me of holidays in the South of France and the Italian Riviera . . .

Ask your fishmonger for a whole sea bass (about 1 kg), gutted, not scaled, with the head left on, but the gills removed and the tail and fins trimmed.

1 whole sea bass, weighing about 1 kg
3–4 fresh bay leaves (optional)
1.6 kg coarse sea salt

to serve
extra virgin olive oil
fresh lemon wedges

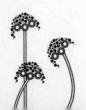

Preheat the oven to 220°C.

Rinse the fish thoroughly in cold water inside and out so that there is no trace of blood. Remove the gills if your fishmonger hasn't already done so (this is very important), then pat dry and season with a little salt in the cavity. Also add the bay leaves, if using.

Choose an ovenproof dish that is big enough to hold the entire fish and spread 400 g of the salt over the base. Lay the fish on top, then pour the remaining salt all over the top of the fish so it is completely covered. Your dish will now look like a baking dish full of salt. Place it, uncovered, in the centre of the oven and bake for 10 minutes for

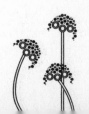

every 450 g, adjusting the baking time
by 5 minutes either way for each 200 g
more or less of fish.

Remove the fish from the oven and let it
stand for 3 minutes to firm the flesh – this
will make it easier to fillet. Brush away as
much salt as possible to prevent it seeping
into the flesh when the skin is removed.
Using a sharp knife, gently scrape the skin
away from the top of the fish. Remove the
bay leaves. Carefully lift off the top fillets,
remove the backbone and then lift the
remaining fillets from the skin. Serve with
olive oil and lemon wedges.

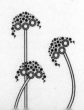

Mixed Fish Coconut Hotpot

If you like, you can add spices to this, such as ground cumin, coriander, chilli and tumeric.

SERVES 6

2 salmon steaks
1 cod fillet, cut into chunks
1 sea bass fillet, cut into chunks
1 carton coconut milk (400 ml)
8 fresh prawns
salt and freshly ground black pepper
1 garlic clove, crushed
1 onion, sliced

Preheat the oven to 180°C. Chop the fish into large chunks and place in a dish with all the other ingredients. Bake in the oven for 25 minutes or until the fish is cooked.

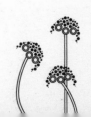

Fast But Healthy

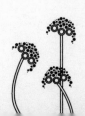

Big O Chicken Burgers

These are a real family favourite, and I always cook more than I think I'm going to need, yet they are always eaten. (The O refers to the fact they are organic.)

4 skinless chicken breast fillets

I teaspoon thyme leaves

small bunch parsley, chopped

I medium onion, roughly chopped

2 garlic cloves, crushed

2 tablespoons tomato ketchup

150 g wholewheat flour

pinch of salt

2 tablespoons coconut oil

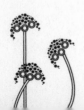

Blitz all the ingredients apart from the flour, salt and coconut oil in a food processor for about 20 seconds, then set aside. Put the salt and all but a tablespoon of the flour in a bowl and scatter the remaining flour on a flat plate.

Wash and dry your hands – we're getting to the messy bit. Take a small handful of the chicken mixture, roll it in the flour and salt until covered, then put it on the floured plate and flatten to a burger shape. Repeat with the rest of the mixture – you should have about eight burgers.

Heat the coconut oil in a large pan and fry the burgers until golden brown on each side. Serve in wholemeal buns with sliced tomatoes, sliced onion and lettuce, and ketchup, mayo and mustard on the side. Yummy.

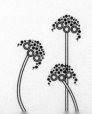

Magic Chicken

Jamie's son Charlie loves this. Although it needs to be left for an hour to marinate, it is incredibly quick to cook. It is particularly nice served with creamed sweetcorn – organic American creamed corn can be found in most Tescos. The quantities given here are enough for two children – or one very greedy one.

1 chicken breast, cut into about a dozen cubes
3 tablespoons maple syrup
2 garlic cloves, peeled and finely chopped
1 medium egg yolk, lightly beaten
250 g plain flour
pinch garlic salt
salt and freshly ground black pepper
1 teaspoon mixed herbs
3 tablespoons olive oil

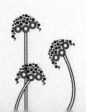

Place the diced chicken in a bowl and add
the maple syrup, garlic and egg yolk. Leave
for an hour to marinate.

Place flour, garlic salt, salt and pepper
and mixed herbs in a large bowl. Dip the
marinated chicken cubes in the flour,
making sure that the surface of the chicken
is completely coated with the flour.

Heat the olive oil in a frying pan and, when
hot, add the chicken and fry until golden
brown. Serve with pasta and creamed corn.

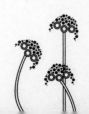

Barbecue Pork Chops

My family loves a good barbecue, especially having seen how the real pros do it in Australia when on tour there. It's a great way to gather the family together in the summer.

4 pork chops
6 tablespoons clear honey
2 tablespoons tomato ketchup
(bought or your own homemade version)
1 chilli pepper, deseeded and finely chopped
1 tablespoon soy sauce

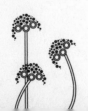

Mix together the honey, ketchup, chilli
pepper and soy sauce and marinate the pork
chops for 1–2 hours before barbecuing.

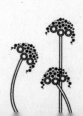

One-pot Wonders

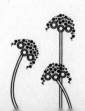

Vegetable Coconut Curry

This is a delicious curry, which I often cook on the road.
If you want to make it hotter, add more chillis.

SERVES 6–8

2 tablespoons olive oil
1 small onion, chopped
3 garlic cloves, crushed
1 tablespoon fresh grated ginger
1 teaspoon mustard seeds
2 teaspoons ground coriander
1 teaspoon ground turmeric
¼ teaspoon cayenne pepper
2 carrots, sliced
200 g string beans, sliced in 2-cm long sections
2 medium onions, sliced
2 green peppers, cut into strips
1 small hot green chilli
250 g flaked, unsweetened creamed coconut

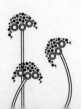

500 ml water
1 ½ teaspoons salt
2 teaspoons sugar
1 pimento pepper, sliced
160 ml natural yoghurt

Heat the oil in a large saucepan, then sauté
the chopped onion, garlic and ginger until
the onion begins to colour. Add the mustard
seeds, coriander, turmeric and cayenne,
and cook for about 2 minutes on a medium
heat. Add the carrots, string beans, sliced
onions, green pepper and chilli. Toss so
that everything is mixed, simmer for a few
minutes, then add the coconut, water, salt
and sugar.
Stir, cover and simmer for 20 minutes.
Remove the lid and let it reduce by half. Stir
in the pimento strips and yoghurt and cook
rapidly for a few minutes.
Taste for seasoning and serve.

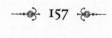

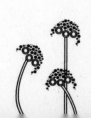

Bubble and Tweak

This is a great leftovers dish and a real favourite with my boys.

4 cooked potatoes (preferably roasted)

2 cooked sweet potatoes

250 g cooked cabbage

125 g cooked peas

250 g cooked carrots

pinch of salt and freshly ground pepper

2 tablespoons HP Sauce

a little olive oil and butter

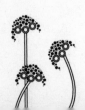

Put all the ingredients in a food processor
and mix for 20 seconds. Heat the olive oil
and butter in a frying pan over a gentle heat,
then spread the mixture across the base of
the pan so you have what looks like a giant
pancake. Cook slowly for 20–30 minutes
without stirring, then, holding a plate over
the top of the bubble, turn it over and slide
it back into the pan to cook the other side.
Continue to cook until the bottom of the
bubble is golden.

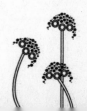

Lentil Shepherd's Pie

This is a great variation of an old favourite.
I make this – and the meat version – regularly.

2 tablespoons olive oil
2 medium onions, chopped
1 garlic clove, crushed
2 tablespoons plain flour
350 ml vegetable stock
1 teaspoon dried thyme
salt and freshly ground black pepper
500 g cooked Puy lentils
600 g mixed vegetables, chopped (use leftovers, cook
some specially or use a packet of frozen mixed veg)
100 g mushrooms, fried
500 g mashed potatoes

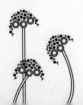

Preheat the oven to 180°C.
Heat the oil in a medium-sized saucepan,
then add the onions and garlic. Cook until
softened, then stir in the flour until it has
been absorbed. Add the stock, thyme,
salt and freshly ground black pepper, and
stir until it comes to the boil. Stir in the
lentils and vegetables, then tip mixture
into a baking dish. Spoon over the mashed
potatoes and bake in the oven for
40 minutes or until browned on top.

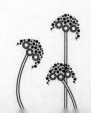

Rock 'n' Roll Stew

I've cooked this many times for our rock 'n' roll friends and I always end up with an empty pot. It's a very filling, healthy and hearty meal.

2 tablespoons olive oil

6 chicken thighs

1 onion, chopped

4 garlic cloves, chopped

2 cm piece fresh ginger, chopped

1 × 400 g can chickpeas, drained and rinsed

1 medium butternut squash,
peeled, deseeded and cut into chunks

125 g orange lentils

2 medium sweet potatoes, peeled and cut into chunks

4 medium carrots, cut into chunks

approx 750 ml chicken stock

pinch of nutmeg

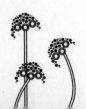

Preheat the oven to 150°C.

Heat the oil in a large pan that can subsequently go in the oven, then add the chicken and brown well. Remove with a slotted spoon and set aside. Add the onion to the pan and cook until tender but not coloured. Add the garlic and ginger and continue to cook for 1 minute. Add the chickpeas, butternut squash, lentils, sweet potatoes and carrots, and season with salt, pepper and a grating of nutmeg. Return the chicken to the pan. Pour over enough stock to cover everything with about 2 cm to spare, cover with a lid, bring to a simmer, then place in the oven for about 1 hour or until the veggies are tender and the chicken is cooked through.

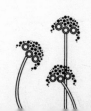

Malaysian Chicken Curry in Coconut Milk

2 tablespoons oil

1 chicken, jointed into two breasts,
two legs and two thighs

2 onions, chopped

3 garlic cloves, chopped

1 teaspoon chilli powder

2 teaspoons curry powder

1 teaspoon paprika

1 teaspoon cumin

1 bay leaf

2 tomatoes, roughly chopped

3–4 tablespoons chopped fresh coriander

450 g sweet potatoes, peeled and cut into chunks

250 ml coconut milk

750 ml water

salt and freshly ground black pepper

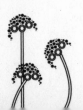

Heat the oil in a large pan and brown the chicken pieces really well. Remove from the pan and set aside. Add the onions to the pan and fry for about 5 minutes until tender but not coloured. Add the garlic and spices and continue to cook for a further minute until the spices are fragrant. Return the chicken to the pan, along with the sweet potatoes, coconut milk and water, and season to taste with salt and pepper. Bring to the boil, cover, and simmer for 20–30 minutes until the vegetables are tender and the chicken is cooked through. Adjust the seasoning and serve.

This is delicious served with steamed rice,
fresh yoghurt and pineapple raita.

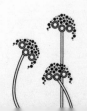

Breast of Chicken Florentine

This was a regular when my kids were teenagers.

700 g spinach

2 tablespoons coconut oil

1–2 pinches ground nutmeg

30 g butter

4 skinless chicken breasts,
preferably with the wing bone still on

salt and freshly ground black pepper

300 ml single cream

1 level teaspoon mild French mustard

100 g Dutch cheese, grated

2 egg yolks

25 g parmesan, freshly grated

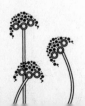

Pick over and wash the spinach in plenty of cold water. Cook in the coconut oil over a low heat until wilted. Add salt and pepper to taste, and a little nutmeg. Arrange the spinach over the base of a flameproof dish and keep warm.

Melt half the butter in a sauté pan until foaming, then brown the chicken on both sides. Season well with salt, pepper and nutmeg. Pour over all but 2 tablespoons of the cream, reduce the heat, and simmer for 5–6 minutes, turning the chicken over halfway through the cooking time. Remove the chicken and place on top of the spinach, then set aside and keep warm.

Boil the cream and butter sauce rapidly for half a minute. Whisk in the mustard, then stir in the cheese and simmer until all the cheese has melted. Mix the egg yolks with remaining 2 tablespoons of cream. Remove the cheese sauce from the heat and whisk in egg and cream mixture. Pour over the chicken breasts, sprinkle with parmesan, then brown under a hot grill.

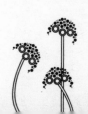

Traditional Irish Stew, with Soda Bread

I cook this traditional dish in Ireland, using lambs raised by our gardener, Patrick. We like it served with soda bread and a green salad.

Irish Stew

1 kg boned lamb or mutton

4 large potatoes

2 large onions

4 large carrots

Salt and freshly ground black pepper

Small bunch parsley, chopped

Water, or stock, which gives a better flavour,

but isn't vital

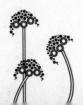

Cut the meat into largish chunks. Peel and slice the potatoes, onions and carrots. Layer the meat and vegetables in a deep pan, starting and ending with potatoes. You will need a deep pan with a tight-fitting lid, or a casserole dish that can go on the top of the stove. Season generously with salt and pepper. Cover with water or stock. Bring slowly to the boil and skim off any scum that comes to the surface. Lower the heat to the merest simmer, cover and leave to cook for about 2–2 ½ hours. Strew over the chopped parsley, just before you serve the stew.

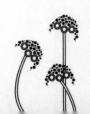

Soda Bread

450 g plain flour
1 tsp salt
1 tsp baking soda
1 tsp sugar (optional)
350 ml buttermilk

Pre-heat your oven to gas mark 8, 450°F, 230°C.

Sieve the flour, salt and baking soda into a
large mixing bowl. Make a well in the centre
and pour in most of the buttermilk – you
may not need the full amount. Mix the flour
and buttermilk with your hand until you

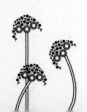

have a dough, adding more milk if needed.
The mixture should not be too wet or
sticky. Turn the dough onto a lightly floured
surface and knead it briefly, forming it into
a round loaf. Put it onto a lightly floured
baking tray and make a cross in the top with
a knife. Soda bread does not need to proof,
just put it straight onto the top shelf of your
oven and bake for about 30 minutes. When
the loaf is cooked, it will sound hollow
when rapped.

Turn it out onto a wire rack and
leave it to cool.

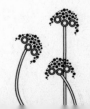

Minced Beef Stew

This is Ronnie's favourite supper.
I make it at least once a week so if he is painting or in
the studio he can heat up a bowl at any time of night!

2 tablespoons olive oil

1 onion, chopped

500 g minced beef

2 teaspoons Marmite

1 tablespoon HP Sauce

1 cup water

2 large carrots, sliced

1 cup peas

8 new potatoes or 4 winter potatoes

salt and freshly ground black pepper

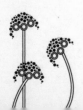

Heat the oil in a large pan and gently cook
the onion until it is translucent. Add the
mince and cook through. Add the Marmite,
HP Sauce, water, carrots, peas and potatoes.
Season with salt and freshly ground black
pepper and cook slowly, covered, on a
low heat for an hour. Add more water
if necessary.

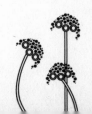

Best Ever Chilli Con Carne

This is nice to spice up those evenings in.

250 g dried red kidney beans or 2 × 410-g cans
kidney beans, drained and rinsed
4 tablespoons vegetable oil
900 g braising steak, cut into 1–2-cm cubes,
excess fat discarded
2 onions, chopped
½–1 teaspoon hot chilli powder or cayenne pepper
1 rounded teaspoon paprika
1 tablespoon cumin seeds
2 tablespoons dark muscovado sugar
3 garlic cloves, crushed
900 g ripe tomatoes, skinned and roughly chopped
600 ml beef or chicken stock
salt and freshly ground black pepper
soured cream or crème fraîche, to serve
roughly chopped fresh coriander, to garnish

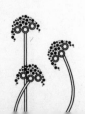

If you're using dried beans, put them in a bowl, cover with plenty of cold water and leave to soak for at least 8 hours, or overnight. Drain the beans and tip into a pan. Cover with fresh water, bring to the boil and boil rapidly for 10 minutes. Drain and set aside.

Heat 2 tablespoons of the oil in a large, heavy-bottomed pan until very hot. Fry half the meat until well browned on all sides. Remove with a slotted spoon and set aside. Repeat with the remaining oil and meat. Add the onions to the pan with the chilli, paprika, cumin and sugar, and fry very gently for 8–10 minutes until deep golden and caramelised. Return the meat to the pan, along with the garlic, tomatoes, stock and drained red kidney beans. (If using canned beans, wait until the last 30 minutes of cooking time before adding.) Bring to the boil, reduce heat and simmer, uncovered, on a very low heat for 1¼ –1½ hours until the meat is so tender it falls apart. Check the seasoning. Serve with a spoonful of soured cream or crème fraiche and garnished with coriander.

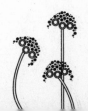

Puddings and Treats

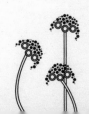

Old English Trifle

I'm not a great fan of puddings myself, but this reminds me of childhood birthday parties, and it always goes down well with the family. Ronnie just loves trifle.

600 ml milk

½ vanilla pod

2 eggs, plus 2 egg yolks

2 level tablespoons caster sugar, plus extra for sprinkling

1 Victoria sandwich cake or 8 trifle sponges

150 g raspberry or strawberry jam

100 g macaroons, lightly crushed

100 ml medium sherry

300 ml double cream

25 g flaked almonds, toasted

50 g glacé cherries

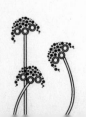

Bring the milk and the vanilla pod to the boil. Remove from the heat, cover, and leave to infuse for 20 minutes. Beat together the eggs, egg yolks and sugar, then strain into the milk, stirring constantly. Cook the custard over a low heat without boiling, stirring until it thickens slightly. Pour into a bowl, lightly sprinkle the surface with sugar and leave to cool.

Spread the sponge cake with the jam. Cut up and place in a 1.5 litre, shallow, serving dish with the macaroons. Spoon over the sherry and leave for 2 hours. Pour over the cold custard. Lightly whip the cream and spread half of it over the custard. Pipe the remaining cream on the top and decorate with almonds and cherries.

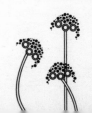

Rhubarb Crumble

Another good, old-fashioned English recipe.
We love it.

10 sticks of rhubarb, cut into 4-cm lengths
100 g caster sugar

for the crumble
200 g plain flour
100 g butter
75 g sugar
pinch of salt

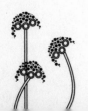

Preheat the oven to 200°C.
Place the rhubarb in an ovenproof dish,
sprinkle with the sugar and mix well. Roast
in the oven for 10–15 minutes or until
tender, then leave to cool. Alternatively, you
can cook the rhubarb with the sugar but no
water in a pan on the stove until soft.

Put all the crumble ingredients in a
food processor and whiz until it has the
appearance of fine breadcrumbs. Spread the
crumble mixture over the fruit and bake for
about half an hour, or until the top is golden.

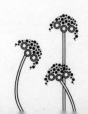

Fresh Fruit Salad

strawberries

blueberries

raspberries

banana

peach

mango

mint leaves

for the syrup

2–3 tablespoons elderflower cordial

juice ½ lemon

2 tablespoons golden syrup

2–3 tablespoons blackberry cordial

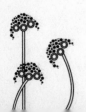

Wash, peel, deseed and chop all the fruit as necessary and place in a bowl. Gently heat the syrup ingredients over a medium heat. When cool, pour over the fruit and refrigerate until required. (It is best to leave for a little while to allow the flavours to develop.)

This is a soft summer fruit salad, so feel free to use any soft fruit that is in season. I haven't given precise quantities as that's up to you.

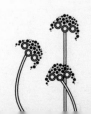

Floating Islands

My mum used to make these for us when I was a child.
This is her recipe.

4 egg whites
60 g icing sugar, sieved on to paper

for the sauce
4 egg yolks
½ teaspoon cornflour
30 g caster sugar, plus extra for dredging
300 ml single cream
1 tablespoon triple-strength rosewater

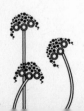

First make the sauce. Cream the egg yolks, cornflour and sugar – in a bowl that can subsequently fit snugly over a pan of simmering water – until light and fluffy. In a non-stick pan, bring the cream to the boil, then pour over the yolk mixture, whisking briskly with a small balloon whisk. Place the bowl over a pan of simmering water and continue whisking gently until the sauce is thicker than single cream but not as thick as double cream. Remove the bowl and immediately stand in cold water to prevent the mixture curdling, continuing to whisk constantly until the mixture is cool.

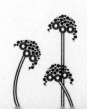

When cool, add the rosewater. Dredge the surface of the sauce with a little caster sugar to prevent a skin forming. Chill well.

To make the islands, whisk the egg whites until stiff peaks form, then whisk in the icing sugar. Fill a shallow pan with water and bring almost to the boil. Using a tablespoon, which should be rinsed in cold water for each new island, spoon four meringue islands (or as many as will fit without crowding) into the water.

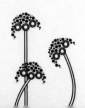

Cook for 3–4 minutes, making sure the egg white is set before turning over each island with a slotted spoon and cooking for a further 3–4 minutes. Drain the islands on a clean towel or kitchen paper and leave to cool. Make the rest and arrange them all in a shallow serving dish. Spoon the sauce over and around the islands and serve.

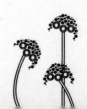

Homemade Chocolate Fudge

Another of my mum's favourites — I remember making this with her as a young girl. It is not for anyone on a diet or who needs to avoid sugar, but it does taste so good. You don't have to add the fruit and nuts.

500 g caster sugar

125 ml milk

160 g cocoa powder

2 tablespoons golden syrup

30 g butter

250 g chopped walnuts or mixed nuts

and fruits (optional)

1 teaspoon vanilla extract

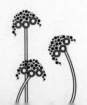

Heat the sugar, milk, cocoa and syrup until the sugar is dissolved. Boil until a soft ball can be formed when a little is dripped into a glass of iced water. Remove from the heat and add the butter, but do not stir. When the mixture has partly cooled, beat until thick and creamy. Add the vanilla, and the nuts, if using, and pour into a buttered pan. When completely cool cut into squares.

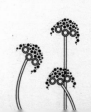

Preserves

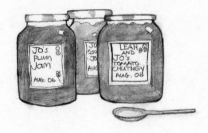

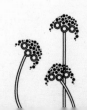

Spiced Ripe Tomato Chutney

makes 1.5–2 kg

1.5 kg ripe tomatoes, roughly chopped

2 medium onions, chopped

2 tablespoons black mustard seeds

2 level teaspoons cumin seeds

2 level teaspoons coriander seeds

1 level teaspoon ground allspice

1 level teaspoon chilli powder or smoked paprika

2 red peppers, deseeded and chopped

2 red chillies, finely chopped

2 garlic cloves, crushed

300 ml malt vinegar

100 g soft brown sugar

75 g raisins

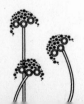

Place the tomatoes and onions in a preserving pan. Toast the spices in a small frying pan set over a low heat for about 1 minute, then add to the tomatoes and onions, along with all the other remaining ingredients. Place over a low to medium heat and allow the sugar to dissolve. Then bring to the boil, reduce to a simmer and cook, stirring occasionally, for 1–1 ½ hours or until the ingredients are soft and almost all of the liquid has evaporated. Pour into sterilised jars, cover and set aside to cool before labelling.

This delicious chutney is best eaten between 2 and 6 months after making, to allow the flavours to mellow.

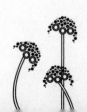

Plum Jam

makes 1.5 kg or 3–4 jars

1 kg plums, washed, stoned and cut into quarters
6 tablespoons water
1 kg preserving sugar

Place the plums in a preserving pan and add
the water. Set the pan over a low to medium
heat and gently simmer until the fruit turns
into a soft pulp. Add the sugar and stir over
a low heat until it has completely dissolved.
Raise the heat and boil until the jam starts
to thicken. To test whether setting point has
been reached, drop a teaspoon of jam on to a
chilled saucer and leave for 30 seconds.

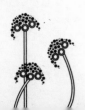

If it wrinkles when pushed with your
finger the jam is ready to be bottled.
If not, continue to cook and test every
3–4 minutes. You could also use a sugar
thermometer to check when the jam reaches
setting point – 110°C. Remove the pan from
the heat and allow to rest for 2 minutes –
this will prevent the pieces of fruit rising to
the top of the jars once bottled. Pour into
sterilised jars, cover immediately and cool
completely before labelling.

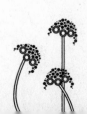

Drinks

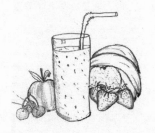

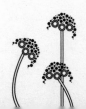

Old-fashioned Lemonade

What could be nicer on an English summer's day?

6 unwaxed lemons

100 ml water

100 g sugar

to serve

iced water or soda water

lemon slices

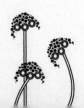

Grate the rind from the lemons, making
sure you take only the yellow zest and not
the white pith, which is bitter. Squeeze the
juice. Pour the water into a large saucepan
and add the sugar. Add the lemon zest and
stir over a gentle heat until the sugar has
dissolved. Boil for a few minutes, then add
the lemon juice. Dilute with iced water or
soda water to taste and serve with ice cubes
and lemon slices.

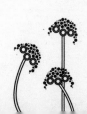

Ginger Beer

2 unwaxed lemons

600 g sugar

1 teaspoon cream of tartar

50 g fresh ginger, peeled and sliced

6 litres boiling water

30 g fresh yeast

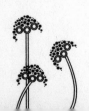

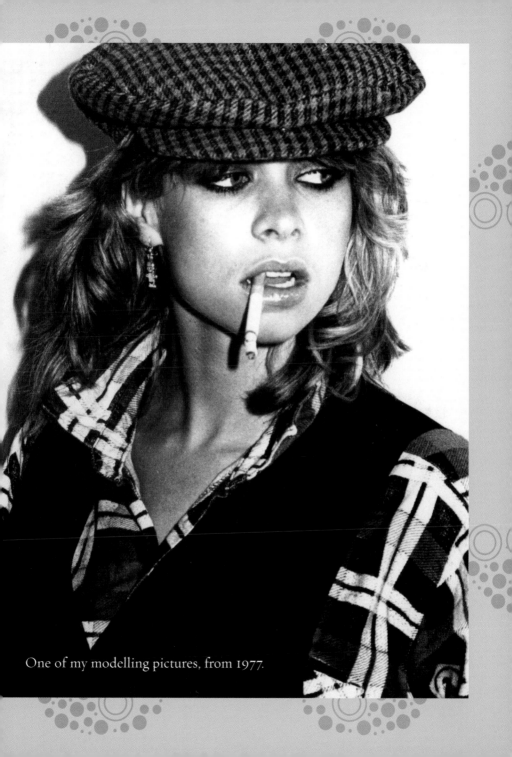

One of my modelling pictures, from 1977.

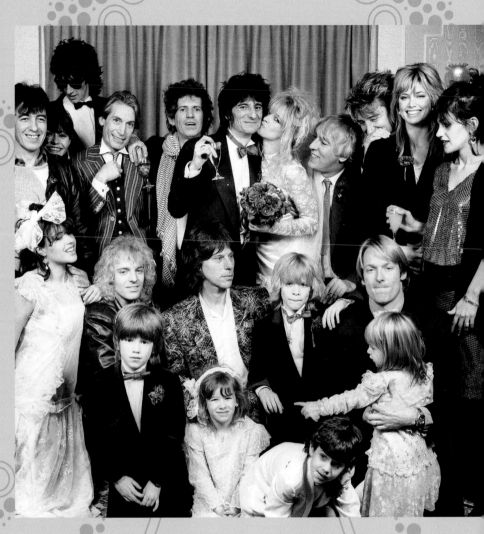

Our wedding – which was a really great party.
Here are Ronnie and myself surrounded by friends and family.

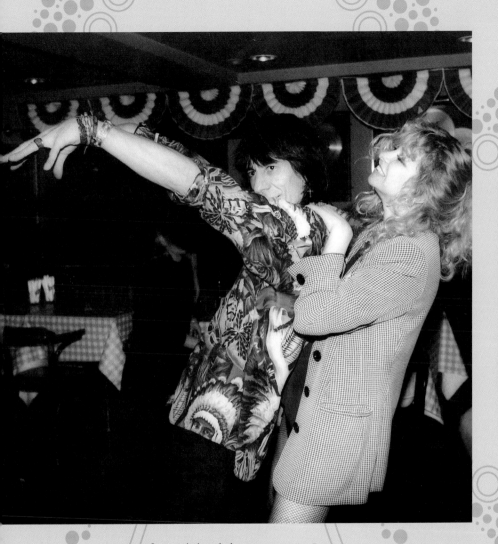

My fortieth birthday, on tour in Japan.

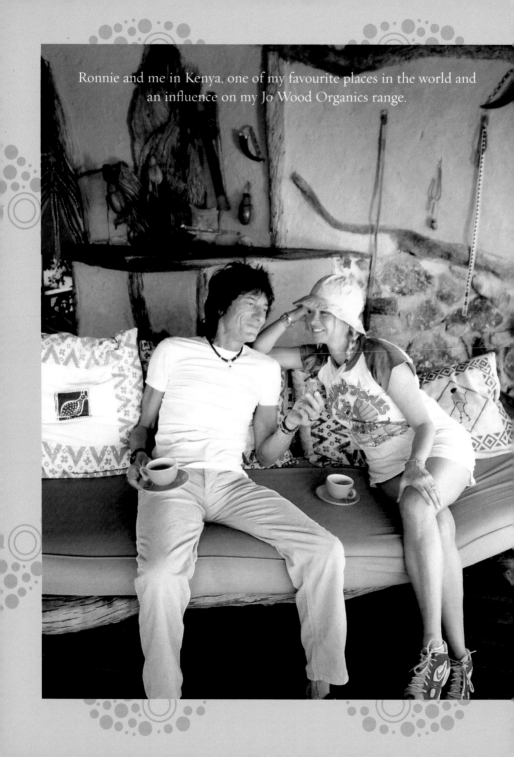

Ronnie and me in Kenya, one of my favourite places in the world and an influence on my Jo Wood Organics range.

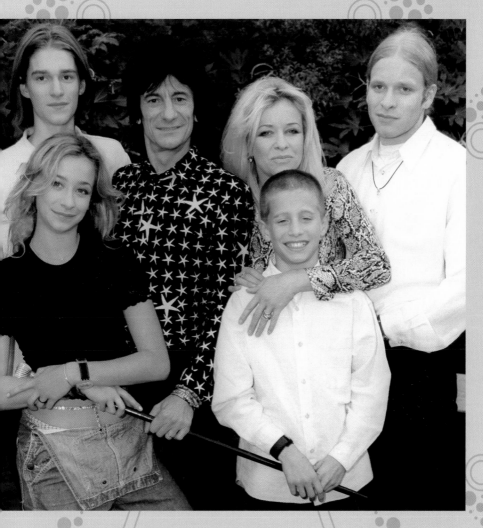

I love this family photo. We were living in Richmond at the time. From left to right: Jesse, Leah, Ronnie, me, Tyrone and Jamie.

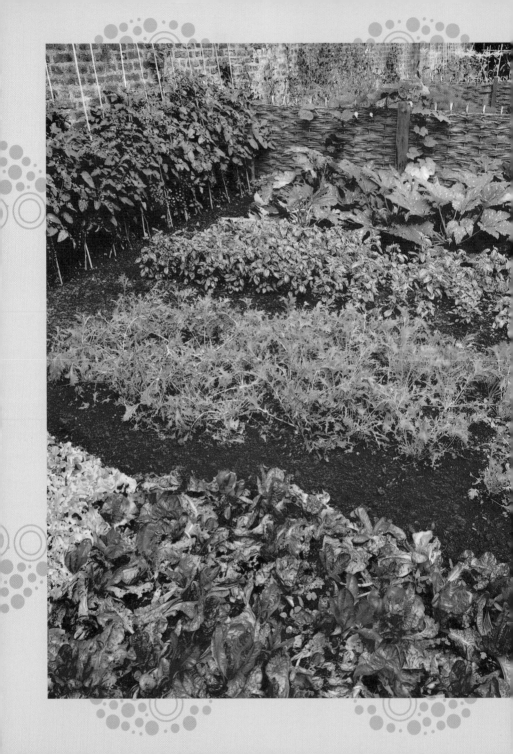

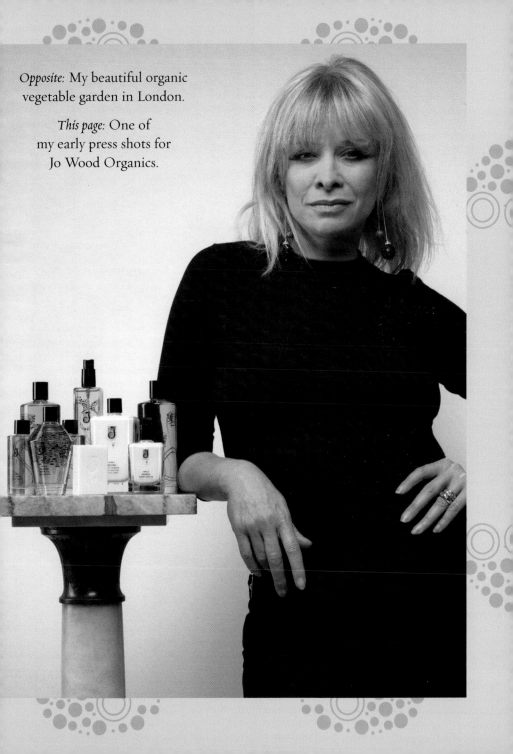

Opposite: My beautiful organic
vegetable garden in London.

This page: One of
my early press shots for
Jo Wood Organics.

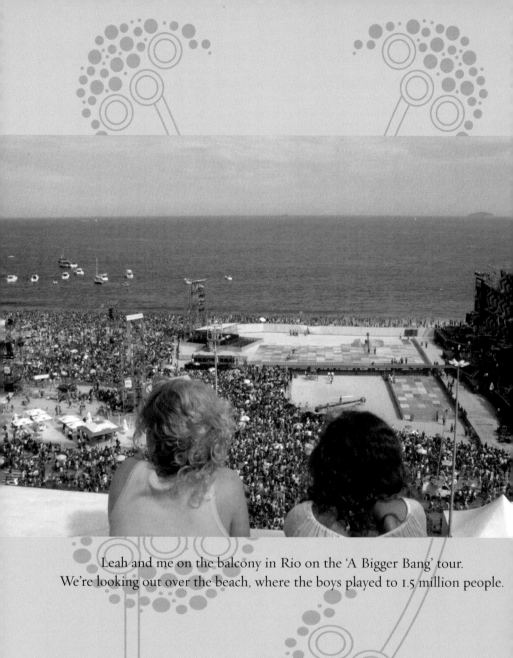

Leah and me on the balcony in Rio on the 'A Bigger Bang' tour.
We're looking out over the beach, where the boys played to 1.5 million people.

Peel the lemons, making sure you remove
every bit of white pith, then slice and
remove any pips. Put the lemon slices into a
large ceramic or earthenware bowl and add
the sugar, cream of tartar and ginger. Pour
over the boiling water and set aside until
it reaches body temperature. Crumble in
the yeast, stir well and cover with a cloth.
Leave in a moderately warm place for 24
hours. Skim the yeast from the top and
strain carefully, watching for sediment,
into bottles. (It may be easier to first strain
into a jug and then pour into bottles.) Seal
with tight-fitting lids. In two days it will
be ready to drink.

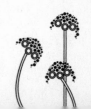

THERAPEUTIC JUICES AND HEALING DRINKS

I love juicing, and I use my juicer daily, whatever the season. I miss it most when I'm on tour, although there are lots of great juice bars around the world these days. I juice whatever I have in my garden, whatever arrives in the organic box – beetroot, celery, carrot – and I love experimenting with different blends. If someone has a particular problem, such as sore gums or a headache, I'll look up the remedy in my nutritional bible and put it in a juice. Like cooking, I just throw in what's available, although there are a few I use regularly. Just add the ingredients below to your juicer and drink immediately – they don't keep.

These recipes are enough for one person.

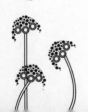

Fijian Splash

This is a delicious juice, great for those suffering from water retention.

small bunch grapes

2 pears

½ melon (any kind), cut into chunks

Turn Up the Volume

This juice is full of antioxidants and bioflavonoids — good for boosting the immune system if you're feeling a bit worn out.

1 pink grapefruit

1 carton cranberries

1 apple

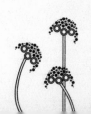

Cool Runnings

A brilliant decongestant for the snuffles. The coriander leaves should be stirred in at the end rather than put in the juicer.

2 carrots

2 oranges

4 tablespoons chopped coriander leaves

No More Catarrh

Soothes the respiratory tract and thins mucus.

2 ripe mangoes

½ lime

300 ml rice milk

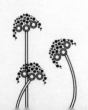

The Morning After

I know this doesn't sound quite as attractive as a bloody Mary, but if you can stomach it, it will make you feel great. The glutamine in cabbage protects the liver against alcohol damage. Again, the coriander leaves should be stirred in at the end, rather than put in the juicer.

¼ cabbage

4 sticks celery

2 teaspoons chopped coriander leaves

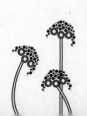

Jo's Detox

*Beetroot is a great detoxer and gets the gut moving;
carrots soothe the lining of the intestine.*

3 large carrots
2 medium-sized beetroots

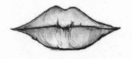

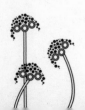

Eye Twinkler

This is a delicious drink, full of nutrients for the eyes.
Children love it too.

2 carrots

2 apples

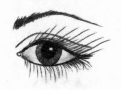

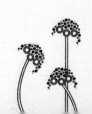

Wake Up Call

This really wakes up your brain in the morning!

4 cardamom pods

2 cinnamon sticks

4 black peppercorns

2 teaspoons grated fresh ginger

600 ml water

1–2 tea bags

50 ml soya milk

honey, to taste

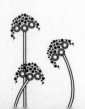

Place the spices in a pan with the water.
Cover and heat without boiling for 20
minutes. Remove from the heat and infuse
the tea bag(s) for 4 minutes. Add the milk
and honey and drink hot.

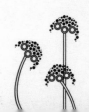

Happy Bunnies

Great for feverish children.
These fruits have antiseptic and decongestant properties.

2 apples, cored and chopped

50 g blackcurrants

450 ml water

2 teaspoons lemon juice

honey, to taste

Place the apple and blackcurrants in a pan with the water and bring to the boil. Simmer for 10 minutes, then strain. Stir in the lemon juice and honey and serve hot.

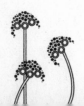

Very Mellow

This is a very good natural antidepressant and tranquilliser.

25 g fresh lemon balm leaves
600 ml boiling water.

Place the lemon balm in a teapot and pour
over the boiling water. Leave to infuse for
10–15 minutes. Drink a maximum of four
cups throughout the day, either hot or cold.

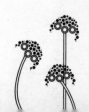

Rock 'n' Roll

This is a first class juice – full of energy and natural zest.

225 g dried apricots

1 teaspoon ground ginger

½ teaspoon ground cinnamon

¼ teaspoon ground nutmeg

½ teaspoon allspice

4 cloves

600 ml ginger ale

½ teaspoon lemon juice

Stew the apricots with the spices in a little water until soft. Blend until smooth, then add the ginger ale and reheat. Add lemon juice to taste and serve.

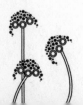

Fab Juices and Smoothies from Planet Organic

Planet Organic is a great store and, as I have mentioned earlier, they have helped us with the bars at our Woodfest parties for many years now. Here is a selection of the juices they have supplied for us in the past.

Planet Zinger ❧ carrot, apple, orange and ginger

The Big Buzz ❧ apple, wheatgrass juice, ginger and ginseng

Super Cleanser ❧ apple, orange, lemon, aloe vera juice

Pear Pleasure ❧ pear, orange, banana and yoghurt

Banananut ❧ banana, almonds, vanilla soya milk

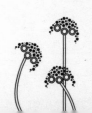

'When I first heard that Jo had gone ORGANIC, eyes raised to heaven, much suppressed chuckling was evident. Some sighed in exasperation. There were quite a few very UNORGANIC jokes. But you have to hand it to the girl, she has won me over, and that ain't easy . . . so GO JO!'

Keith Richards

Part 2

Your Face and Body

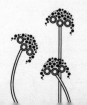

6

Natural Beauty

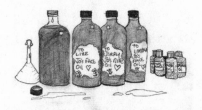

ONCE I STARTED SHOPPING FOR ORGANIC food and reading around the subject, I began to look at the other stuff I used in my home. It was all very well deciding not to eat another chemical, but I was still exposing myself to them in the form of lotions, creams and cosmetics. It has been estimated that women put more than 200 different kinds of chemicals on their skin every day, a staggering number of which are potentially harmful and are thought not only to disrupt hormones but are known to be carcinogenic in animals. The degree to which they are harmful to humans is not yet clear, although there is anecdotal evidence that some products cause allergic reactions, dizziness, headaches and nausea.

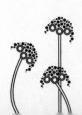

Your Face and Body

In order to make our bodies clean and smooth, and our hair shiny and beautiful, all sorts of terrible chemicals are put into attractive-looking bottles and packages. Some we breathe in, others we absorb through our skin – about 60 per cent enter our bloodstream in this way. Just as we absorb nicotine, hormones or angina drugs from skin patches, so chemicals can worm their way into our bodies. We even lather them on our babies. By law, products have to list the contents on the packaging, albeit in teeny weeny print, and sometimes on a leaflet if the product is too small. The largest percentages are listed first. Unbelievably, there is no legislation preventing companies from using the word 'organic' on products that contain only a tiny percentage of organic ingredients. Nor do they have to list pesticide residues in plant extracts. Even if they did, I suspect we would not know what to make of the strange-sounding compounds.

Once I started doing a bit of research, I became intrigued by what exactly was meant by the term 'natural'. I discovered that there is no accepted, legal definition – which means, in effect, that manufacturers can pretty much say what they like. We need to wise up to the spin on packaging: products can claim to be natural even if they contain less than 1 per cent of natural ingredients! As for hypoallergenic creams, I suspect they are often just the same

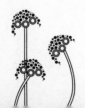

as the regular version, just minus a few colours and fragrances – which, it is true, can cause allergic reactions – but so can many other ingredients. Fragrance is added to nearly everything: not just soap and bathroom cleaner, but cars, paper and even toys. These fragrances are sometimes made of natural ingredients; more usually, they are a potent mix of chemicals artificially combined in a lab to mimic natural scents.

I became fanatical about reading labels. I discovered that particularly nasty substances are often preceded by the word 'contains'. We tend to read these notices as positive features – 'Ooh, look, this contains fluoride. It must be good.' Don't be fooled. I came across a few specialist books that explained these active ingredients and what they do to our bodies, and they confirmed my worst fears. I quickly came to the conclusion that what I should be looking for was products without the following ingredients. This is not a comprehensive list, but I have tried to highlight the most common and the most dangerous.

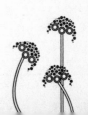

Artificial Colours and Fragrances 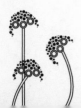 Both can irritate your skin and cause allergic reactions. Synthetic fragrances (which can consist of up to 100 different ingredients) are the biggest cause of allergies to cosmetics. Some colours have been linked with hyperactivity and attention deficit disorder.

DEA (Diethanolamine) Also known as MEA or TEA – look for the initials connected to the ingredient, for example cocamide DEA or stearamide MEA. This is an emulsifier used in lotions, shampoos and creams to create a creamy texture and make them foam. It is not harmful in itself but can react with other chemicals in the cosmetic formula to create nitrosodiethanolamine (NDEA) which is linked to cancer in animals.

Fluoride Unbelievably, it has never been safety-tested on humans, yet in some parts of the country it is still added to our water supply as well as being added to many toothpastes as it helps prevent dental caries. Fluoride does occur naturally – in tea, for instance, in fish and some drinking water. In large amounts it damages bones and enamel, is not recommended in pregnancy and is unsuitable for babies. It has been linked with

irritable bowel syndrome, cancer, arthritis and osteoporosis.
It may help reduce plaque, but so does good dental hygiene.

Formaldehyde 💀 Yes, I thought this wasn't used any more either.
A volatile organic compound, it can still be found in products
such as shampoos, handwash, deodorants and nail varnish.
It is a carcinogen and can trigger asthma.

Lanolin 💀 It sounds nice and natural, and it is an oily substance
extracted from sheep's wool. It can be found in lipsticks and
other oily cosmetics. Unfortunately it can contain traces of
sheep dip. Not nice.

Mineral Oil 💀 This is a sly one. It makes your baby's skin feel
lovely and smooth, it soothes chapped lips and makes your
body feel soft after a bath. Personally, I don't like the idea of
using something that is made from crude oil, particularly as
it can block the pores and dry out the skin.

Parabens 💀 These are chemical preservatives. Some studies have
linked them with breast cancer and infertility, although others
have offered conflicting results. You can recognise them by

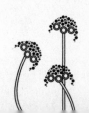

their prefixes methyl- and propyl- etc. They are very widely used in lotions, shampoos, conditioners, hair gels, skin creams, some deodorants, foundations and nail creams. Even baby products include them.

PEG compounds ☠ These may be listed as polyethylene, polyethylene glycol, polyoxyethylene, PEG-6, PEG-150 and are used as foaming agents, humectants and emulsifiers in a wide range of cosmetic products. As part of their manufacturing process, a toxic chemical called 1,4-dioxane can be created, which can irritate the skin, cause headaches and damage the liver and kidneys. PEG compounds can also include small amounts of ethylene oxide which is carcinogenic.

Phthalates ☠ Pronounced 'tarlates', these petrochemicals should be shunned. They are thought to be 'hormone disrupters', which means they can cause fertility problems and affect the development of foetuses. You will find them in lipstick, hairspray and nail varnish.

Sodium Lauryl Sulphate (SLS) ☠ This is the biggie. It is a degreasing agent that is used to make products bubbly and

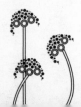

you'll find it almost everywhere, particularly in cheap products. It damages the skin, the wonderful barrier which protects our organs, by removing the hydrolipid, thus allowing other substances, such as dangerous parabens, to go through easily. SLS, and its less harsh alcohol derivative, Sodium Laureth Sulphate (SLES), has been linked with skin dryness and irritation, fertility problems, and damage to organs and our immune system. Japanese studies suggested that SLS may be a mutagen, in other words a substance that causes cells to mutate. It can also react with other chemicals to produce cancer-causing nitrates. Scientists insist that in tiny quantities it is safe, but personally I'm not prepared to take that risk.

Deodorants and Anti-perspirants 🕱 Deodorants have come under the spotlight recently due to parabens, which some contain, having been found in breast tumours taken from women with breast cancer. I think this is more than just one of those scare stories that regularly do the rounds. Parabens can mimic the behaviour of oestrogen, and it is oestrogen that causes tumours to grow. Many anti-perspirants also contain aluminium, which works by blocking the sweat pores. Aluminium is a neurotoxin associated with Alzheimers disease. Look for natural

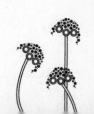

deodorants that are paraben- and aluminium-free. Do not buy antiperspirants: the lymph nodes under our arms are designed to eliminate toxins through perspiration. If you block them, the toxins have to go somewhere else . . .

I knew I had to find alternatives. Some of the new organic stores were, thankfully, waking up to consumers like me and starting to sell products that avoided many of these ingredients. I soon realised it wasn't enough for products to be labelled organic, they needed to be certified too. Being certified means that the manufacturers have had to conform to certain criteria (which have been changed and updated over the past decade). The Soil Association, for example, now requires the maximum amount of organic and the minimum amount of synthetic ingredients. Ingredients must not be harmful to health and they must cause minimum environmental damage. If a product is labelled organic, it must contain a minimum of 95 per cent organic ingredients. If it has less than that, it can still be certified as long as it has at least 70 per cent organic materials and states the percentage on the packaging. Any non-organic ingredients must be non-GM and can only be used if the organic version is not yet available or is one of a limited range of synthetic materials that have been proved to have no harmful effects. There are other bodies

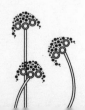

besides the Soil Association, such as Ecocert in France, and I'm pleased to say all these organisations are starting to work together on a common European organic beauty and cosmetic standard.

I was looking for bath oils, body lotions, perfumes and moisturisers. I did find some creams and lotions, and I used them for years before developing my own products. You'll find information on organic ranges at the back of this book. It's best to try a range and see what appeals to you.

I looked for organic make-up too. I'm not a great consumer of make-up – I find foundation clogs my pores – but, again, it was (and still is) incredibly hard to find chemical-free mascara and eyeliner. I thought about dyeing my eyelashes, but I discovered that the dye is worse for you than bleach. (Hair dyes can affect some people very badly, giving them a terrible rash.) There weren't any organic perfumes at all. Today, there are a few organic make-up ranges available – I'm currently trying the Lavera range – and I'm sure we'll see big developments in this area over the next few years.

Knowing this, my brother gave me a book he thought I would be interested in, *The Fragrant Pharmacy*. Inspired, I started mixing my own essential oils, making up potions for myself and my family with organic oils I ordered from a specialist supplier. I used oils as moisturisers, with different blends for day and night. In the same

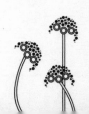

way that I relish experimenting in the kitchen, I found I adored trying out different blends and remedies. I became fascinated by the therapeutic qualities of different oils, and I loved the way some of the smells reminded me of the exotic places I had visited with Ronnie. I bought some little glass bottles and made up special blends as gifts for friends.

ESSENTIAL OILS

Essential oils should never be applied to your skin in an undiluted form, and you should always check with your doctor or a qualified aromatherapist before using them if you are pregnant, have asthma, epilepsy or are on medication.

There are many ways in which these wonderful oils can be used, below are just a few suggestions:

🦢 Add 6–12 drops to the water in a burner to fragrance a room.

🏵 Mix 3–5 drops into a teaspoon of base oil and swirl them into a warm bath.

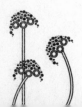

Use as a massage oil. For just one massage, add 2–4 drops to 10 ml (a tablespoon) of base oil. If you want to make up a bottle, add 15–30 drops to 100 ml of base oil.

There are lots of base oils, which in themselves have therapeutic properties. The following are the most widely available:

Grapeseed Non-greasy, it is suitable for all skin types.

Jojoba Rich in vitamin E and excellent for all skin types.

Peach Kernel Particularly good for facial blends, as it is easily absorbed. Contains vitamin A.

Sweet Almond Full of vitamins and minerals, and a good base oil for massage. Works for all skin types, but is especially good for dry skin.

Wheatgerm Rich in vitamin E and good for mature or dry skin.

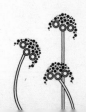

My Favourite Essential Oils

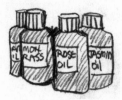

These organic essential oils are the first ones I ordered in when I started making blends in my bathroom.

Bergamot ᴗ Widely used by aromatherapists to treat depression, relieve stress and insomnia, bergamot is balancing, reviving and refreshing. The oil is extracted from the bergamot fruit, which resembles a small orange.

Cardamom ᴗ Sweet and spicy, cardamom oil is good for the digestion, warming to the senses, refreshing and uplifting.

Cedarwood ᴗ From cedar trees grown in Morocco, this oil is calming and soothing. Its deeply woody aroma contributes to the base note of both of my organic fragrances and is particularly appealing to men.

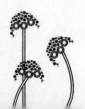

Natural Beauty

Clary Sage ✑ A herbal, citrusy and slightly nutty fragrance, clary sage is known to ease nervous tension, a racing mind and is deeply relaxing and warming.

Clove ✑ Clove's strong, spicy aroma has a positive and stimulating effect on the mind. It is known to strengthen memory and has wonderful uplifting qualities when you are feeling weak, lethargic or depressed.

Coriander ✑ With a warm sweet aroma, coriander has a stimulating, refreshing effect on the mind, especially when you are feeling lethargic, nervous or tense.

Galbanum ✑ Derived from a shrub found in the Middle East, galbanum has a musky aroma evocative of damp woodlands. It has a grounding effect and can calm erratic moods and ease nervous tension.

Geranium ✑ Sweet smelling, a little like rose with minty overtones, geranium quells anxiety and depression and lifts the spirits.

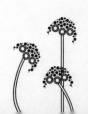

Ginger ✧ Hot ginger's aroma is spicy and sharp with a hint of lemon and pepper. It warms the emotions when feeling cold or tired. It is also stimulating, sharpens the mind and aids memory.

Guaiacwood ✧ Deep, strong and earthy with smoky vanilla undertones, guaiacwood has a deeply relaxing effect, aids meditation and helps relieve nervous tension.

Jasmine ✧ Heady and sweet, jasmine is a flowery, exotic oil. It is a valuable remedy for depression as it's calming to the nerves, warming to the emotions and produces positive feelings of confidence.

Mandarin ✧ Bright, fresh and fruity, the aroma of mandarin oil is intensely uplifting and can help to banish anxiety.

Neroli ✧ Uplifting and restorative, neroli's citrusy aroma acts as an antidepressant and helps soothe and calm the mind.

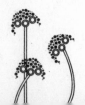

Natural Beauty

Palmarosa ✣ Organically grown in Nepal, palmarosa has a calming yet uplifting effect on the emotions. It is also said to refresh and clarify the mind.

Patchouli ✣ With a strong, earthy, exotic aroma, tempered by a sweet spiciness, patchouli is believed to be a mild aphrodisiac. Its aroma promotes a balancing and grounding effect, which helps banish lethargy and sharpen the wits.

Petitgrain ✣ Obtained from the leaves and twigs of the bitter orange tree, petitgrain's aroma is uplifting and balancing and helps to relieve tension, fatigue and stress.

Pineneedle ✣ The pineneedle oil in my range is derived from Scottish pine trees and has a strong, fresh, forest fragrance. It is stimulating and refreshing for tired minds and general feelings of weakness and lethargy.

Rose Otto ✣ A symbol of beauty and love, rose otto oil has a deep, sweet, flowery aroma. It has a soothing effect on the emotions, lifting the heart and easing nervous tension and stress.

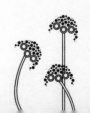

Rosemary ~ Invigorating and refreshing, rosemary is good for mental strength, relieving general dullness and lethargy.

Vetiver ~ Vetiver (also called Vetivert) is derived from a wild grass grown in the Far East and India and has a deep, smoky, earthy fragrance. It is intensely calming, emotionally strengthening and settles the nerves to bring about a sense of balance.

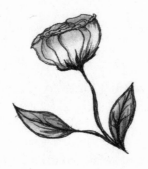

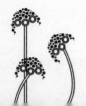

AROMATHERAPY BLENDS

Here are some lovely aromatherapy blends to soothe both the mind and the body using oils that are readily available. They should be added to 25 ml of base oil.

To Aid Digestive Problems

5 drops black pepper
4 drops orange
4 drops peppermint

or

5 drops basil
3 drops peppermint
4 drops camomile

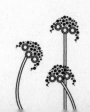

To Relieve Aches and Pains

5 drops ginger
4 drops lavender
3 drops marjoram

To Ease Stress

4 drops frankincense
4 drops bergamot
3 drops neroli

or

5 drops clary sage
4 drops ylang-ylang
3 drops cedarwood

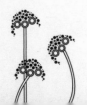

To Bestow Calm and Confidence

6 drops bergamot
3 drops peppermint
3 drops lavender

To Cheer You Up and Clear Your Head

5 drops cardamom
3 drops grapefruit
3 drops lemon

or

6 drops cypress
4 drops rose
2 drops frankincense

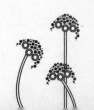

Your Face and Body

To Ease Anxiety

5 drops cedarwood
2 drops lemon
2 drops geranium

or

4 drops patchouli
3 drops neroli
2 drops nutmeg

To Relieve Hot Flushes and Menstrual Cramps

7 drops cypress
3 drops clary sage
2 drops geranium

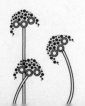

To Calm Children's Tantrums

2 drops camomile
2 drops mandarin
2 drops lavender

Sensual, Romantic Blends

4 drops rose
3 drops neroli
3 drops frankincense

or

3 drops ylang-ylang
3 drops jasmine
3 drops vetiver

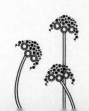

My Beauty Routine

*'The human face is the organic
seat of beauty.'*

Leah Wood

Now that I have my own range of beauty products I am often asked what my own beauty regime is. I am always tempted to say SMILE. It makes everyone look young and full of life. I keep a laughing Buddha on my dressing table to remind me of this. You always have a choice, and the conscious brain can only hold one thought at a time. Choose a positive thought.

But back to the question, what I do is very simple. First thing in the morning I not only brush my teeth but also my tongue. Sounds slightly unpleasant, I know, but it is a great thing to do. Not only does this give it a good clean, scraping off a layer of bacteria, it also sends a wake-up message to the gastric juices, telling them to get ready to digest food. Have a good look at your tongue. If it has a

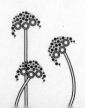

nasty white coating on it you know you overdid it the night before – it's basically a sign of toxins, either food or drink. If that's the case, have a light breakfast.

Then I brush my body with a special body mitten I got in Toronto. You can find similar ones, made out of sisal or hemp, in health food shops or you can use a brush. I do this every day, taking it slowly, working up from the soles of my feet, using circular movements, and always brushing towards the heart. It helps the lymphatic system remove toxins, and makes you tingle all over. It's good for cellulite too.

I follow this with a steam in my steam room, but, if I'm on tour, a hot shower will do, followed by a cold shower. Once in the steam, I use a salt scrub rather than soap. This is a great exfoliant and really wakes up the circulation, as well as making your skin feel very soft. I follow this by moisturising with oil or lotion (my own, of course). Afterwards I put one of my own oil blends on my face and a moisturiser.

While I'm getting dressed, I'll sip hot water with half a lemon squeezed into it – great for a fresh, clean feeling and a healthy digestion. It keeps my skin blemish-free, too. Then for breakfast I'll usually have goat's yoghurt with honey and wheat-free toast, washed down with green tea. I take my vitamins regularly and Cellfood

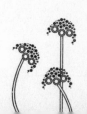

drops (which supply oxygen, minerals, amino acids and enzymes). If I'm feeling under the weather I take 2,000 mg vitamin C. During the day I make sure I drink a glass of water every hour – water is vital for clear skin, clear thinking, and a million essential unseen tasks carried out by every cell of our bodies.

Before I go to bed I always take off my make-up with organic or natural make-up remover. I'm always trying out new ones, researching what is available until one day I can hopefully bring out my own. I'm trying out facial scrubs too, as I'm also developing a face range. The final step is to moisturise.

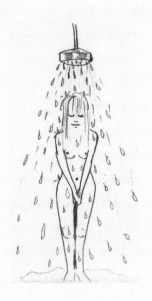

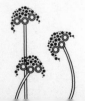

Face Masks and Body Scrubs

It's easy and fun to make your own face masks and body scrubs – these are a few recipes to get you started.

Avocado and Egg Mask ᔫ A lovely moisturising treat. Blend an egg white with the flesh of a whole avocado and 1 teaspoon lemon juice. Smooth over the face and neck and relax for 20 minutes. Rinse off with a mixture of milk and water.

Honey Mask ᔫ Organic honey is a natural antiseptic and this mask is fantastic for removing dead cells and impurities. Mix together 2 tablespoons clear honey and 1 tablespoon almond oil. Apply over the face and neck, massaging in for 3 minutes. Relax for 20 minutes, then rinse off with warm water.

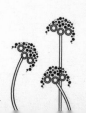

Wheatgerm Cleansing Scrub ᴧ A refreshing, bracing
scrub that will leave your skin glowing with health.
Warm 7–8 tablespoons milk, pour into a bowl,
then add 8 tablespoons wheatgerm, stirring until
you have a paste. Massage into the skin, paying
particular attention to any dry or rough areas.
Rinse off with tepid water.

Oatmeal, Almond and Lemon Cleansing Scrub ᴧ Suitable
for all skin types, this one smells delicious too. Mix
together 2 tablespoons fine oatmeal, 2 tablespoons
ground almonds and 2 tablespoons grated zest
with a fork, and add a little water to form a paste.
Massage into the skin using circular movements,
always working towards your heart. Rinse off with
tepid water.

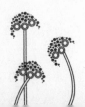

7

My Own Line

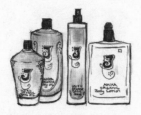

ONE DAY JAMIE SAID, 'Mum: all these bottles you keep mixing up for people – you should be selling them.'

'My own line? What, professionally? Don't be silly, too much like hard work!'

'You'd love it.'

'I wouldn't know where to start.'

And we left it at that, but I did start to think. Ronnie was drinking quite a bit around this time, and I found I was spending far too much time worrying about him. One day, when I must have been looking particularly exhausted, my mum said to me, 'You've

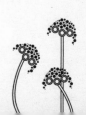

spent your life looking after other people, Josephine. It's about time you found yourself a hobby.'

'That's all very well for you to say, Mum. But what?'

'I don't know, that's for you to decide. Find something you're passionate about.'

'Confucius said, "If you are not happy you must make yourself happy. It is easier to wear a pair of slippers yourself than to try and carpet the whole world."'

Rachel Karslake (Jo's mum)

Then someone asked me to go in with him on an organic venture, and I suddenly realised my name might have some currency. This got me thinking even more. One evening I'd just got back home, laden with shopping, and was cooking supper when I thought to myself, Mum's right. Leah was out with her lovely boyfriend, Jack. Ty was off with his mates. Ronnie was painting. I'm just the one

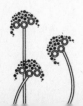

that does the cooking. And they don't even need me to do that any more. I realised that the time had come for me to follow my own passions. So I shoved the casserole into the oven and went and did an hour's yoga. When I had finished I felt calm and strong. I knew I was going to develop my own products. And once I'd decided, that was it.

Later that night, Ronnie was dismissive. 'You'll never get that together.'

'Thanks,' I said. And I thought, I'll show him. Once I am challenged, I always rise to the bait.

The more I thought about it, the more excited I got. I tried the idea out on friends, most of whom thought I wasn't being serious, until I went on and on about it. Many people tried to put me off. One acquaintance said, 'Be very careful, Jo. Lots of rock stars' wives think they can start a business on the back of who they are. You have money, glamour, great connections – but it doesn't mean you are going to be successful.'

None of which deterred me. First I sat down with Donna and Emily, two good friends who work with us in the office, and discussed the how, who, what and when. Next I sat down with Jamie, and discussed the idea from all angles. Nothing put me off, I was excited and determined to do something positive. I had a lot

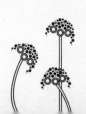

of knowledge about organic living. I knew about upscale products. I was certain there was a gap in the market for sophisticated, organic body products. There was nothing I had seen on the market that was luxurious enough for me or my bathroom shelf. If this was true for me, then I was sure it was true for others.

'Let's do it, Jamie!' I said, all fired up. I was determined that my passions would become a reality. 'It will be a luxury range that smells gorgeous and is organic too. I'm going to do it, and I'm going to do it properly.'

I had lunch with a good friend, Jo Fairley, who gave me a few pointers and told me to call Colette Haydon. Colette is a very experienced French cosmetologist who has worked with many top companies in making up perfumes, and she would be able, according to Jo, to help me make up two or three fragrances that could then be made up into body products. So I called her, and not long afterwards we sat down in her laboratory and I told her what I wanted: a range of products that were not only organic and pure, but that would smell different from the existing ones on the market, and look chic. In other words something new and unique. She was great and immediately understood where I was coming from. I was overjoyed.

I babbled on about what I saw as a gap in the market, described some of the blends I had made up myself, and the kind of scents

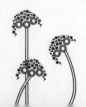

I loved. I talked about the importance of organic products from food to toiletries. The more I talked, the more confident I felt. Particularly as she was nodding in agreement.

'My work is not just about helping you to decide on the smells that go into a particular fragrance,' she said in strongly accented English. 'I try to put into a product something of your personality. So I have to get to know you and together we will work on formulating something very sophisticated, very sexy, something divine.'

She talked some more about the process of putting fragrances together, and I knew I would be able to work with her. She is clever, thoughtful and passionate about her work – quite a character, in fact.

To kick off with, she asked me to write a list of all the scents I like. I thought about the flowers I grow in my garden to bring the fragrance of spring and summer into the house: jasmine, gardenia, lavender, hyacinths. About the freshness of lemon and the tang of vetiver, a scent used in men's cologne. Then I thought about how leather and smoke and patchouli always bring to mind those hazy rock 'n' roll nights. How oriental scents such as cinnamon and cloves recall days wandering through eastern markets and watching the dawn come up in the southern hemisphere. I have travelled so widely – India, Thailand, Japan and Africa – I wondered if there was a way to capture the spirit of the exotic places I had been to.

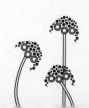

There were so many scents I adored – how on earth were we going to make something out of all of them?

I showed my list to Colette and she laughed.

'But this is you all over! Very interesting combinations. How much do you want to be involved in the process of refining the fragrances?'

'I want to be involved in every step,' I replied. 'How can I put my name to something if I haven't had anything to do with it?'

So that was how we started. We would meet every week, mixing and blending essential oils together in Colette's laboratory, experimenting with different percentages of each oil. I learnt that each blend needed top notes, middle notes and base notes. ('Just like music,' commented Ronnie wryly.) These blends would be added to a vegetable oil, known as the 'base', and every week or so I would have a new one to take home and try out on Ronnie and the kids. I was astonished at how different they all were, even though we were using only four or five oils. We must have tried out hundreds of different combinations. I easily rejected many of them for being too strong, too medicinal, too floral, too spicy, too insipid. I wanted two or three separate fragrances, and the challenge was to find smells that were both different *and* gorgeous.

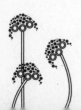

'Jo is a woman of many contrasting elements, and this is expressed in the fragrances she loves. She is drawn to floral scents and citrus scents; she likes to mix oriental notes with floral scents. It is very unusual, this desire to mix a fragrance with its opposite. But if I think about Jo's life, I can see how she has lived with the glamour and excitement and the exposure, but at the same time she is intensely private, and a very homely, motherly person.'

Dr Colette Haydon

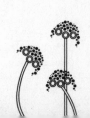

The ones I was particularly drawn to tended to be fragrances rich in smoky, woody notes: sandalwood, cedarwood, rosewood. I knew one of the final perfumes would inevitably be a musky, 'woody' one. We joked about this, of course, because of my surname – how appropriate! The other one to emerge was more citrusy – a lighter fragrance with a refreshing tang.

When, finally, I was happy with the initial blends, we went to a perfumer. This is the crucial next stage, which ensures that a fragrance is 'stable' or long lasting. To our minutely described fragrances the perfumer added tiny amounts of certain other essential oils to 'harmonise' them. Quantities of concentrated perfume were then passed to the factory. Again, I was involved in every step.

Although vital to the final product, deciding on the scents I liked was only a tiny part of the whole process. Over a period of nearly two years, we were not only working on the mixture for the base product itself, but simultaneously talking to suppliers and perfumers, working with designers on the packaging, visiting the factory, discussing launch plans, distribution, marketing and publicity, and – most importantly – researching the organic dos and don'ts. We contacted the Soil Association in order to establish what rules and regulations covered the production of fragrances and body products. They are, of course, the best-known and most authoritative body on organic

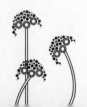

farming and food production and only lend their stamp of approval to fully certified organic products. When we went to see them they were just starting to turn their attention to cosmetics and toiletries, and I like to think we helped them as much as they helped us, for their rules changed during the period we were working with them.

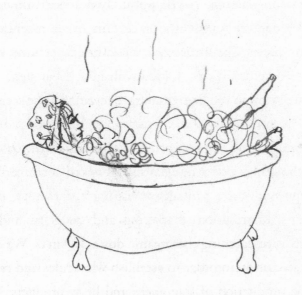

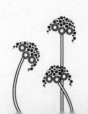

Your Face and Body

It was an incredibly complicated process and, in our determin-
ation to be as organic as we possibly could, we reformulated and
reformulated until we got our products as near perfect as possible.
We researched the sources of organic essential oils, and discovered
that they were not terribly easy to come by. Merely choosing 'natural'
fragrance compounds is not enough: they are not permitted, as the
plants may have been sprayed with pesticides. At one point we had
to reject certain oils ('absolutes') that were extracted using a solvent,
in case there were still traces of the solvent remaining in the finished
product. We had to reject other oils that were produced from
endangered species. We had to find a factory that would conform
to the Soil Association's regulations, and so it went on. All the
way along we worked to their guidelines, until we faced a shortage
problem. The crucial decision came when we could not obtain
enough organic neroli for a test run. What if that happened again
and I had thousands of bottles waiting to be filled and placed into
boxes printed with the SA logo? Some African farms, for example,
that produce wild neroli do not spray their crops but are not *officially*
certified organic because of the high cost of doing so. We couldn't,
therefore, use their crop *and* conform to the SA requirements. In
the end, we realised we had no option but to go ahead without
the official SA symbol, knowing that we were creating gorgeous

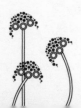

products that contained the highest possible percentage of certified organic ingredients, but that, in the event of a shortage, we would go for uncertified organic. At the back of the book you'll find more information on our organic aims. I believe the SA guidelines are still being refined and developed. As far as organic body products and cosmetics go, the rules and regulations are now where food was fifteen years ago and I hope in the future there will be more organic suppliers and we won't have this problem.

Life is full of setbacks. SUCCESS is determined by how you handle them.

THE JO WOOD ORGANICS RANGE

The Jo Wood Organic Range contains my favourite essential oils, as listed on page 231. The products also include the following ingredients, all of which, I thought you'd be interested to learn, have additional therapeutic benefits.

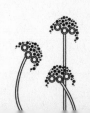

Apricot Kernel Oil ∿ A light, easily absorbed oil extracted from crushed apricot kernels. It has nourishing and moisturising properties, acts as a barrier against moisture loss and is particularly good for those with dry or sensitive skin.

Arctic Bilberry Seed Oil ∿ An extremely rare and very expensive oil extracted from wild Arctic bilberries. Native to the Arctic region, these berries are rich in essential fatty acids and vitamin E, both nutrients essential in regulating the moisture and sensitivity of skin. Packed full of energy and vitality, Arctic bilberries have extremely high levels of antioxidants, which help the body fight damaging free radicals.

Arnica ∿ A soothing, anti-inflammatory herb, commonly used to treat skin disorders, it is also an excellent anti-decongestant.

Calendula ∿ A calming and anti-inflammatory herbal extract, calendula helps to heal and repair the skin.

Carrot Extract ∿ Rich in vitamin A, carrot extract encourages cell division and collagen formation, and rejuvenates tired skin.

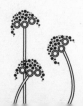

My Own Line

Cocoa Butter ✑ Made from the roasted seeds of the cocoa tree, cocoa butter is an excellent moisturiser and helps improve skin barrier function against moisture loss.

Echinacea ✑ This herb is well known for its immune-boosting qualities, but it is also a powerful anti-inflammatory ingredient and helps promote cell renewal. When combined with St John's Wort in several of our products it helps reduce skin redness or irritation.

Evening Primrose Oil ✑ Hydrating and replenishing, evening primrose oil is great for dry skin, restoring suppleness and elasticity. Rich in essential fatty acids, it encourages collagen formation and helps to reduce skin inflammation.

Ginkgo ✑ Taken from the gingko biloba tree, an ancient tree grown in China, ginkgo has mildly anti-inflammatory properties and helps boost circulation.

Ginseng Extract ✑ Known as an energy booster and tonic, ginseng helps to regenerate and revive by boosting blood circulation,

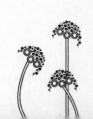

enabling increased supply of oxygen and nutrients and encouraging the elimination of toxins.

Grapeseed Oil ᚙ Containing powerful antioxidants, this highly effective oil protects the skin against damaging free radicals.

Guarana Extract ᚙ Extracted from a small bean grown predominantly in South America, guarana is an excellent tonic for tired heavy legs, as it boosts circulation in the capillaries, increasing the flow of oxygen and nutrients and encouraging the elimination of toxins.

Jojoba Oil ᚙ A highly effective, soothing moisturiser, jojoba helps to boost skin lipid content and improve skin barrier function against moisture loss. Closely resembling the skin's own sebum, it is suitable for all skin types.

Mexican Honey ᚙ Organically produced in Mexico, honey is purifying and soothing, it reduces bacterial contamination and any associated skin irritation.

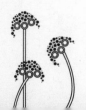

Oatmeal ᔕ Oatmeal is known for its anti-inflammatory and immune-boosting properties. It soothes the skin and reduces any redness or irritation.

Orange Water ᔕ This unique and dynamic ingredient, extracted from organically grown Italian oranges, is the very purest form of vegetal water. Rich in trace elements, and closely resembling the water in our skin, it is an excellent transporter of nutrients right to the heart of the skin's cells. This increases vitality and boosts collagen formation, which improves skin tone and firmness.

Rosehip Seed Oil ᔕ Packed full of vitamins and known for its healing properties, rosehip seed oil is rich in essential fatty acids, which help to regenerate skin cells and encourage collagen formation.

Shea Butter ᔕ Derived from the fruit of the African karite tree, shea butter is soothing and moisturising, and is particularly effective for dry skin.

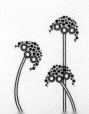

Soybean Oil ✒ Rich in phospholipids, a natural liposome, soybean oil boosts skin lipid content and improves the penetration of natural actives.

St John's Wort ✒ Containing many beneficial properties, St John's Wort is well known for its uplifting properties, and is particularly useful when you're feeling down or poorly. It helps soothe, heal and repair the skin and, combined with echinacea in several of our products, it helps reduce skin redness or irritation.

Vine Extract ✒ A powerful antioxidant that protects the skin against free radical damage.

I won't pretend that the process wasn't without its frustrations. There were moments when I felt we would never get there, that my goal of making divine organic fragrances was simply unattainable. Colette and I would start the week feeling fresh and positive, but by Wednesday morning we would have had a setback of some kind, and by Friday we would be pulling our hair out in desperation. On one occasion, organic cocoa butter was nowhere to be found as it was Valentine's Day and it had all been requisitioned for luxury

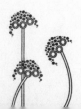

chocolates. Another significant problem was the need to include water in the body lotion and body dew. If we were to fulfil the organic criteria we couldn't use the usual filtered or distilled water. First, I came up with the idea of aloe water, then Colette went one better.

'We will use organic oranges,' she announced. 'This ultra organic fruit water comes from Italy, the oranges are filtered until the water is in the purest form.'

This sounded fab to me, though I had never heard of such water. 'What about the expense?' I asked.

'If we want to be truly organic, this is our water.'

And so it was that we ordered our organic filtered orange water from Italy. Later, we were pleased to discover that this orange water, known as vegetal water, actually had additional antioxidant health benefits. This made the extra cost a little easier to bear. I had already reconciled myself to the fact that my products were going to be expensive: organic essential oils are twice the price of non-organic oils, and natural oils are ten times more expensive than those synthetically produced in a laboratory to mimic natural fragrances.

When I was briefing the design team, having finally found a company who understood where I was coming from, I explained that the containers had to be glass, because it was a naturally derived

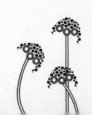

substance and was recyclable. I had already chosen the bottles, each one a different shape – echoing my collection of antique scent bottles at home – because I knew I wanted to have a different design for each category. These products were organic, but I wanted them to look sexy. I wanted the range to be eclectic, to be reminiscent of the Biba look I had so loved in my early modelling days, and I wanted an Art Nouveau influence. I was also drawn to the raunchiness of black and gold. I was obsessed with detail – nothing was going to be left to chance. And it paid off. I am thrilled with the final look, and the gloriously curvy 'J' that adorns all the bottles.

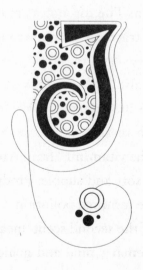

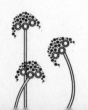

So in the end we got there. Two wonderful fragrances – one bright and fresh, the other sensual and woody. Both come in a lotion, body oil, bath oil, body soap and body dew. I gave them Swahili names because they remind me of Africa, a place full of scents that arouse the senses: the wild flowers and tropical seas, and the scent of the savannah at dusk. We always go on holiday with ALL the family once a year (when not on tour), to Kenya. I really love Africa and feel very at home there. Ronnie and I help raise money for the Tusk Trust, to help save the elephants and the rhinos.

Amka, the name of the first scent, means 'to wake'. It is designed to be refreshing after a long flight, or to pep you up before a night out on the town. The top notes are neroli and bergamot, the heart notes are extracts of Iranian rose otto and Egyptian jasmine, and the cedarwood base has traces of green mandarin and sweet oranges. It also has extracts of guarana, ginseng and gingko – these all boost the circulation. The apricot and grapeseed oils it contains are rich in antioxidants and protect skin against free radical damage. The vitamin E, from Arctic bilberry seed oil, leaves the skin feeling soft and supple. Products from the Arctic are very pure due to the minimal pollution.

Usiku, the name of the second scent, means 'night' in Swahili. The top notes are rosemary, pine and guaicwood, with a touch

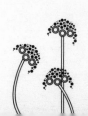

of cardamom and hot ginger. Middle notes are made up of spicy coriander and cloves with cleansing clary sage. The base notes are Moroccan cedarwood, patchouli and vetiver. It also contains arnica, echinacea, calendula and St John's Wort. This is the 'woody' fragrance. It is much mellower than Amka, and I like wearing it when the weather is cooler, as it is a really warm fragrance.

Just before the launch of my products, which was held in London at shopping heaven Harvey Nichols in October 2005, I said to Ronnie, in a told-you-so kind of voice, 'You thought I'd never do it, yet here we are. I did it!'

'Nah,' he said, 'I only said that to wind you up. I knew you'd want to prove me wrong.'

Here, at last, was my organic range, and I was so proud of myself. It was chic, sophisticated and smelt divine. But, best of all, it has no petroleum derivatives, mineral oils, sodium laureth sulphates, parabens, phthalates or other chemically derived active ingredients. There are no genetically modified ingredients, and all organic ingredients come from accredited and audited sources. The most brilliant thing about having these products, though, is it has given me a great reason to get out there and talk about my passion for living organically.

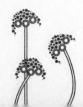

I am continually working with the Jo Wood Organics team on developing new products for my range. We also work with our suppliers to try and increase the supply and demand for organic ingredients to make them more widely available. This is so important.

Jo is one of those people who was born young – which to me is about looking good, happy and sexy, whatever your age. Her fragrances are very daring, very rock 'n' roll. They are a reflection of her eccentric personality.

Dr Colette Haydon

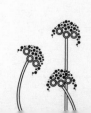

Developing these products has been a fantastic learning curve for me. At first I was so shy and awkward having to deal with professional people in industries I was unfamiliar with, and I realised I had spent too long in the shadow of other people. Gradually, as I learnt more about what we were doing, I became more confident, and I started to develop my own opinions. Where once I was tongue-tied in meetings, I now find it so easy to talk. I know what I think, I know what I want, and I'm entirely happy in my own skin.

It's helped my marriage, too. Now, if Ronnie has a drink, I'm not consumed with worry for days. I'm too busy! I accept that it is his problem, and that I can't continuously be nagging him. A few years ago, he went on the wagon and did a whole tour without drinking, which was truly brilliant. Then he started dabbling, knocking back a little shot here and there. Then soon he was back drinking and it was driving me nuts. I even left him for a while, checking into Champneys health spa, sticking a note to the fridge that said, 'I'll come back when the real Ronnie is back.' I wasn't going to leave him for ever – after all, I married him for better or worse. But I wanted to shock him into changing. It didn't work, of course. I love him dearly and I would be delighted to have him clean and sober, but at long last I have realised that I can't take someone else's addictions on my shoulders. He wouldn't want me

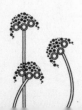

to, anyway. He has an on-going battle with booze, and I'm realistic about that. Alcoholics don't get better, it's a constant struggle. I know he thinks about his addiction all the time. Last New Year's Eve, he said, 'I'm giving up smoking.' And I was able to reply, calmly and sincerely, 'Good. I hope you succeed.'

While I was working on this book, Ronnie went back into rehab, and since then he's been doing great. It can be a bit of a roller coaster, though. Life goes back to normal for a while and it's lovely, until he has a drink again and it all goes to pieces. I know people out there whose partners won't go into rehab at all, so I admire him so much for continuing to try. Every time I hope against hope that it is going to last more than a few weeks or months. If he could put a year behind him that would be fantastic: I know he really wants to succeed.

Sometimes now I get home and think, wow, I haven't given Ronnie's problems a thought all day – how fantastic! Starting my own business has been the greatest. I was told at the therapy sessions in Arizona and London, that the best thing to do was to look after No.1 – me – and that has really worked.

I am often asked what keeps us together, and I think that mostly the answer is patience. I was born with lots of it. Plus we fit well together – I'm a good listener, and he loves to talk about

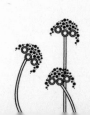

himself! I was prepared to give up my career and be the one doing the looking after. There was a moment when I thought I'd like to be an actress – in fact I told Graham Chapman at one of our New Year's Eve parties that that's what I wanted to be and the next week he put me up for a part in a film about rehab. I loved the experience of five weeks on location, but was happy to get back to my role of wife and mother. I love Ronnie as much as I did when we first got together twenty-eight years ago; more, in fact, because of all we have been through together. I understand his weaknesses and I admire his willingness to try to deal with his addictions, I love listening to him play guitar and I love watching him paint. When he is sober he is pure genius. But it can be very hard work, living with His Majesty.

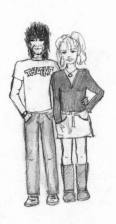

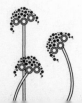

My Own Line

There are those men born to sorrow and despair

And those men born to a woman with a good pair

There are those men born that are lucky in life

And those men born that have a fab wife

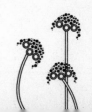

8

Exercise and Relaxation

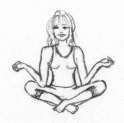

Exercise and relaxation are as essential to outward beauty as they are to inner beauty. We need exercise for a strong, healthy body and sweating once a day is important to regenerate your skin. The glow that comes from exercising your muscles, and doing something *for yourself* is better than any number of facials. Relaxation is important too: it allows your mind and body to recharge and let go of anxieties and problems. Try to get into the habit of including 20 minutes of quiet contemplation in your day, even if it is only sitting on a park bench at lunchtime or having a long soak before bedtime. It really does make a difference.

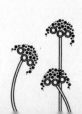

Your Face and Body

There are lots of ways to get exercise into your life – swimming, joining an exercise class, just walking – but these are some of my favourites.

YOGA

Yoga was one of those things I'd been aware of for years, but had always associated with old Indian guys getting themselves into impossible positions. It wasn't until 1988 that I thought I'd try it for myself. My first experience was with my sister and good friend, Lorraine. We went to a yoga class in Notting Hill, but it wasn't a huge success. The teacher was young, handsome and extremely flexible. All he had on were tiny short shorts and, as I stood in the tree pose, he stood right in front of me and asked, 'And what's your name?' All I could do, I'm afraid, was giggle uncontrollably.

Luckily, I found Tina, who's been my teacher now for five years. Yoga is one of those things you can read about, you can even look up positions in books and try to follow them, but there is no real substitute for having a good teacher. Tina is so chilled; she has a great body, even though she is a bit older than me, and she totally understood what I was trying to achieve.

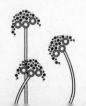

Exercise and Relaxation

I found yoga fitted in perfectly with my new, clean life. It's all about being calm, about living well and in harmony with the universe, about respecting your body and the planet. It works on a physical level, it works on the mind and emotions, and it also opens up a spiritual dimension.

I started gradually, but soon I was on to three sessions a week with my teacher, plus whatever I could do by myself at home. I noticed myself becoming more relaxed, less tense, more aware of my own needs, and more confident that I could deal with all the conflicting pressures of life. Now I feel very committed, focused and determined. I love to do yoga and try to do it three times a week. I wish I had more time on the road to do yoga – that's when I could really do with it!

There are various different styles of yoga, and the one that I was attracted to most is called Sivananda, which was brought to the west by Swami Vishnu Devananda some thirty years ago – around about the time I met Ronnie, in fact. The focus is on the postures and breathing, and you'll often hear it referred to as Hatha yoga. It helps people develop concentration and control of their mind to improve physical health. This appealed to me, because it seemed like a natural accompaniment to my efforts to eat a better diet.

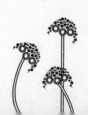

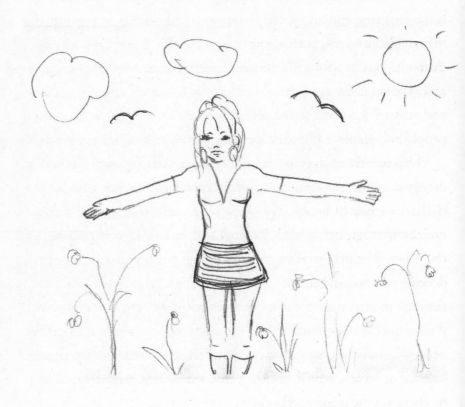

Breathe. It lets you live in the moment.

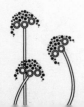

Exercise and Relaxation

My classes start with breathing exercises, move on through some postures, and end with meditation. I like the slow, rhythmical movements, and the fact that because some of the postures are quite difficult it takes effort and concentration. I like moving into a pose and holding it for some time, feeling the loosening up of my joints and muscles. I like the fact that the postures are named after animals, people and plants – it reminds me that we are all interconnected.

The breathing exercise at the beginning of a yoga session is designed to bring you into the present moment. The one I like to do is alternate nostril breathing. Believe it or not, our bodies naturally breathe through one nostril for around two hours, then transfer to the other. The pressures of modern living, however, mean that this delicate process can become unbalanced. Yogis believe that to breathe through the left nostril for too long can lead to chronic fatigue and illness, and to breathe through the right for too long can lead to nervous conditions. So the aim of the exercise is to restore the natural balance of breath, which in turn balances the sides of the brain and re-energises the mind and body.

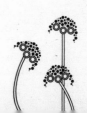

Alternate Nostril Breathing

1 Place your right thumb over your right nostril and inhale for four counts.

2 In a swift movement close your left nostril with your right ring finger and little finger, while removing your thumb from the right nostril, and exhale through this nostril for eight counts.

3 Inhale through the right nostril to the count of four seconds. Close the right nostril with your right thumb and exhale through the left nostril to the count of eight seconds.

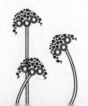

This is called one round. When I started, I used to do it three times, but now I do six to ten rounds. Even if I haven't got a yoga class I find it's a great thing to do first thing in the morning. Of course, if you've got a bad cold don't even think about it!

Do yoga so you can remain active in physical sports as you age.

Since I have been following this regime, my circulation has improved drastically – my feet used to go blue with cold when I first started the *asanas* or postures. I'm sure it has also helped me give up smoking. More than that, I now have an inner strength and a much clearer sense of who I am.

Yoga has taught me why my mum used to tell me to take a deep breath if I was angry or upset about something. Breathing exercises are an essential part of yoga. Breath is the flow of energy that draws the life force into our bodies and is seen in yoga as the link between our bodies and mind. Once you become aware of your breathing using the special yoga techniques your mind stills and you feel healed and energised. Normally we only use a small percentage of

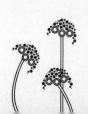

our lungs' capacity; with yogic breathing you learn to take in the maximum amount of air, which sends life-giving oxygen zooming to all the cells in your body.

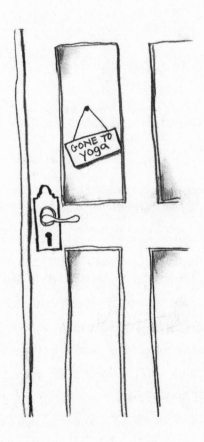

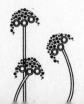

Breathing to Relax

This exercise will make you feel relaxed and calm.

🐝 Lie flat on your back, legs 60 cm apart, with your arms at an angle of about 45 degrees, palms upwards. Close your eyes.

❀ Focus your mind on your breath, feeling your abdomen rise and fall.

🐝 Count while you breathe – in for four, hold for one, exhale to the count of eight; inhale for four, hold for two, exhale for eight; inhale for four, hold for three, exhale for eight. Continue the progression until you are inhaling for four, holding for eight and exhaling for eight.

❀ Let your normal breathing return and notice how calm you feel.

🐝 Flutter your eyes open.

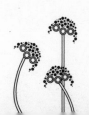

Tibetan Rejuvenating Exercises

These simple exercises are what I do when we're on tour. I can do them in my hotel room, or in the gym or on the beach. It is thought that these exercises work on the *chakras*, or centres of energy, to stimulate the endocrine system, keeping you healthy and young.

The goal is to be able to repeat each exercise 21 times, but to start with you may want to try three repetitions and increase them as you get stronger.

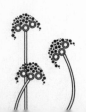

1. Stand upright, extend your arms at shoulder
   level, palms down, and spin clockwise. Keep
   your eyes staring ahead but don't focus
   on any point, allow your vision to blur.
   Keep going for 21 spins (but stop sooner if
   you feel dizzy). When you stop spinning,
   breathe deeply from your stomach until your
   head stops
   spinning and
   your balance
   returns to
   normal.

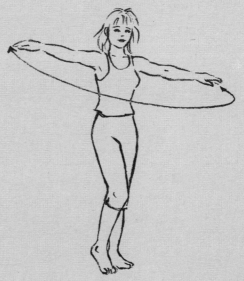

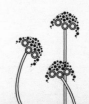

2. Lie down on your back with your arms to the side, palms up. Breathe slowly and raise your legs off the ground as high as you can. Then raise your head off the ground, bending your neck so your chin falls towards your chest.

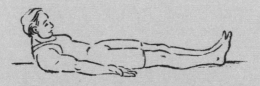

Exhale and relax as you lower your legs and neck. It will take some time for your tummy muscles to have strengthened enough to do this as many as 21 times, but that is the ultimate goal.

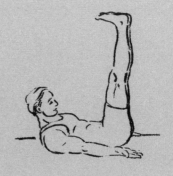

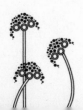

3. Kneel with your legs together, arms out in front of you, palms facing your thighs. Drop your chin to your chest and start to inhale. Raise your head and lean back. Move your hands to the back of your thighs and let them drop lower to support your weight. Drop your head back and relax your spine. Begin to exhale as you return to the starting position.

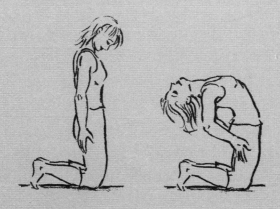

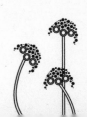

4. Sit on the floor, legs shoulder width apart, arms at your sides, hands flat on the ground, fingers pointed forward, and drop your head down. As you begin to inhale, raise your buttocks off the ground while bending your knees, and shifting your weight to your arms/hands and legs/feet. Continue to raise your buttocks until your body and thighs are parallel to the ground, then let your head fall back. Tense all your muscles, then let them relax as you begin to exhale and return slowly to the starting position. You should rest before repeating this exercise.

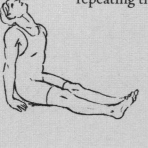

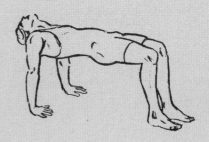

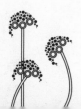

5. Get down on the floor on your hands and knees, as if you were doing a press up. Begin to inhale, come up on your toes, allowing the weight to rest on your arms, straighten your legs, arch your back and lean your head back. Only your toes and hands should touch the floor. Start to exhale as you bend at the waist and push your buttocks up into the air, making an upside down V shape with your arms and legs straight. Tuck your chin under and try to put your feet flat on the ground. Begin the next inhalation and repeat up to 21 times.

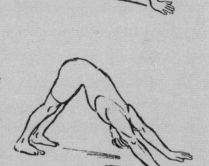

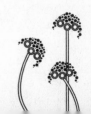

To finish, lie face down on the ground, arms outstretched. Close your eyes and wait for your heartbeat to return to normal.

The ability to relax properly is something that has come to me over time, and yoga has helped enormously with this. I used to think that flopping in front of the telly with a glass of wine and a joint was the best way to wind down. But, if you think about it, we only relax fully when neither the mind nor the body is using up any energy. Only then are they able to recharge. Stress, stimulation, worry, busyness – all these use up energy and leave us feeling tense. It's not just starting my own business that has taken my mind off other stresses, it has been my new-found knowledge that, within myself, I have the tools to calm my exhausted mind.

These tools are the ability to perform controlled postures, to breathe deeply and consciously, and – the ultimate goal of yoga – to meditate. My teacher tells me that meditation slows the rate at which our bodies decline – so it helps keep you young and beautiful too!

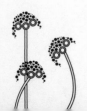

Exercise and Relaxation

MEDITATION

Meditation is a state of mind in which you consciously still all the jabbering and chattering in your mind, all the noise and hustle and bustle, and just *be*. The aim is to be aware only of being in the present. If you can achieve this – or even come close – it's a great way of de-stressing. Studies have shown it reduces blood pressure, relieves chronic pain and can even help overcome substance abuse. It's pretty difficult, particularly if you live in a house like mine, where there is constant bustle, loud music, kids coming and going, grandchildren shrieking, dogs barking, laughter – the thousand different sounds that make up our days and crowd in on our consciousness. It does take lots of practice to still your thoughts completely, but I'm gradually getting better at it, and I feel more serene as a result.

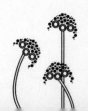

Successful Meditation

Following these tips will help you achieve more successful meditation.

🐝 Decide on a regular time and quiet place to do your meditation – first thing in the morning or last thing at night is best.

✿ Set up a small table with an image or symbol that will help you focus – a flower, a candle, a stone: something simple.

🐝 Sit with your legs crossed, palms on each knee, thumb and middle finger touching.

✿ Hold your back and neck straight.

🐝 Start with a few minutes of deep breathing, gradually slowing your breath so you become aware

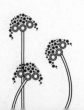

of your breathing. Inhale through your nose for a count of three, then exhale through your mouth for a count of five.

❀ Ask your mind to be quiet, let it wander if it must, but keep bringing it back.

❀ Be aware of your surroundings, but do not allow yourself to react to them.

❀ Focus your attention inwards, on a spot inside your body.

❀ Repeat, if you wish, a mantra, such as OM, which helps stop your mind wandering.

❀ Meditate for ten minutes a day, increasing to an hour over time.

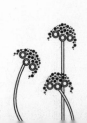

Chakra Meditation

Eastern mystics believe that everyone has an astral body (not to be confused with the soul). Inside this astral body are seven *chakras,* or centres of energy. The *chakras* are connected to the physical body by the meridian system, which you can imagine as a series of tubes. These in turn are connected to the body's endocrine system. If the *chakras* are working efficiently, then the endocrine system functions well. If they aren't, you will feel fatigued and listless. By doing this exercise you help balance the *chakras* and bring them into alignment. It should leave you feeling calm and energised.

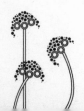

- Sit with your eyes closed, turn your focus to the base *chakra*, situated at the base of your spine. Visualise the colour red for 3–4 breaths.

- Move your mind's eye up to the pelvic area to the sacral *chakra*. Visualise the colour orange for 3–4 breaths.

- Move to your navel, where your solar plexus is. Visualise the colour yellow for 3–4 breaths.

- Move up to your heart and visualise the colour green for 3–4 breaths.

- Next concentrate on your throat *chakra*. Visualise the colour blue for 3–4 breaths.

- Move to the space behind your closed eyes. This is your third-eye *chakra*, and the colour to visualise is indigo.

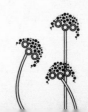

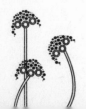 Turn to the top of your head, the crown *chakra*. The colour to visualise is violet.

🌼 Return now to whichever *chakra* seems to call to you. Spend a few moments breathing gently and visualising that colour.

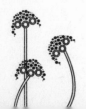 Flutter your eyes open, stretch and notice how you feel.

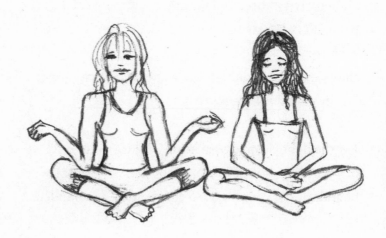

Ball of Light Healing Exercise

This exercise is based on the ancient technique whereby you imagine yourself in the centre of a ball of divine light.

Sit quietly, eyes closed, and imagine a huge bright star above you. It radiates loving, living light. Feel the light streaming over you and invite it to enter the top of your head and pour down through your body, cleansing it as it streams down, carrying away all negativity, disease, fear and tiredness. Focus particularly on washing any part of you that hurts with the bright light. As the darkness washes out of the soles of your feet, see it being absorbed by the kindly earth and being turned to compost.

Let the light cleanse your heart, and fill every cell of your body. It is so bright that it bursts out of the boundaries of your body, so that you are surrounded

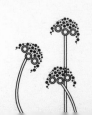

by a ball of healing, protective light. Tell yourself that all positive thoughts from others will penetrate the ball and reach you, but all negative and destructive elements will bounce back, with a blessing returned to the sender.

If you are inspired to try yoga yourself, you'll find hundreds of courses, centres and books. I started yoga because I thought it would tone my body in a way that didn't involve sweating in a gym. I have achieved a toned body, but I've also found so much more. There is a great deal of research now into the positive benefits of yoga on mind/body health and its ability to slow down the ageing process. I firmly hope that, like those old Indian guys, I'll be doing yoga well into my eighties.

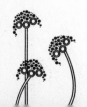

PILATES

Named after Joseph Pilates who invented it, this is a system of precise exercises that appear to be gentle, in that they won't get your heart racing, but that actually have a profound effect on your muscles. The exercises come from a variety of different disciplines such as dance, boxing, gymnastics, yoga and body building. The aim is to realign your spine, the key to health and flexibility. Practised regularly, Pilates will help you feel and look great – even in jeans. It gives you a tight bum, flat tummy and toned thighs – what more could a girl want?

The idea behind Pilates is that our bodies are defined by the way we move, sit and walk, and by the repeated daily actions we do without a second thought. Think how you slump over the computer, strain your back picking up your children, lounge in front of the television, or sit awkwardly in bed reading. Over time these movements become ingrained habits and we develop strengths and weaknesses in different areas, depending on these different stresses (not to mention the effects of gravity and age). The result is an imbalance in your whole body.

Pilates exercises are designed to restore your body's balance by strengthening the muscles of your trunk, abdominals, lower back,

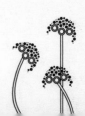

hips, inner thighs and buttocks. They also make you very aware of your posture, retraining you to move in different ways, so as not to put undue pressure on areas that can't handle it. You'll find that, with practice, you will use the easy, fluid movements of Pilates when carrying out everyday tasks such as cooking, driving or running upstairs.

As with yoga, breathing and concentration are vital, as is learning relaxation techniques. However, unlike yoga, where the positions can seem impossible without years of practice, the positions taught in Pilates look – and are – do-able.

EXERCISE

My recipe for a good workout involves:

Balance, poise and control.

Making sure I take my spine through its four main movements: flexion, extension, rotation, and lateral flexion (side bending).

Working up a sweat and feeling the release of endorphins.

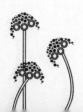

—◌ 294 ◌—

I find my body moves more freely and more naturally using a combination of all of these. Depending on my level of energy, the group of exercises I choose for my workout will be either flexibility-based or strength-based, but each exercise must work the spine. Then to balance my workout I always work on alignment and movement around the pelvis, as well as freeing and balancing the shoulders. It will come as no surprise to you, then, to hear that for my workouts I have chosen a trainer who adopts a holistic approach — what he calls 'structural integration'. He aims to build muscle strength through fluidity of movement and correct posture, rather than strength through tension — as you'd find in a standard gym workout. The aim is to strengthen and realign the core skeletal muscles: those across the back, shoulders, abdominals, 'glutes' and inner thighs. His approach combines yoga and Pilates, as well as elements of fitness training. I start my workout with a five-minute warm-up on the treadmill, or out on my bike to the nearby park if the weather is warm. I'll then work through a series of postures and weight-bearing moves based on yoga and Pilates. We don't use weights, just the weight of my body as resistance. I do five minutes of gentle postures, alternating with five minutes of intense aerobic exercise until my heart rate is 175 beats per minute. I see my trainer between one and three times a week, depending

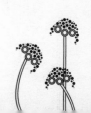

on my schedule, and the sessions last an hour. If I'm on tour, then it's the hotel gym for me. Whatever combination of exercises I do, and wherever I am, I know that my body is in good enough shape to allow me to deal with whatever life throws at me.

You may feel it's too expensive to have a personal trainer, but I can really recommend it. Sometimes, whatever our good intentions, when it comes to it, the motivation just isn't there, but if you've booked a regular session with a personal trainer you're less likely to decide to watch telly instead! And a trainer can tailor an exercise regime for your particular needs. You can always get together with a group of friends to book a trainer and share the cost or, if you're a member of a gym, they may well offer you a trainer as part of the package.

An hour of aerobic exercise releases endorphins to regenerate cells and offset stress.

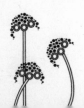

MASSAGE

It sounds like a luxury, and I do realise that many people feel they don't have either the time or the money to head off to a spa or therapy rooms and lie in bliss for an hour or so being massaged and soothed. I've got so much to do! They cry. Some of you may even feel it is too intimate an experience to strip off down to your undies in front of a stranger and have them lay their hands on you.

In fact, unless you have high blood pressure or are particularly ill, in which case you should avoid it, massage can be very beneficial for many aches and pains, headaches and injuries. It also makes you feel relaxed and ready for anything. It works by increasing lymphatic circulation, which aids the release of waste products, and by softening scar tissue and by encouraging oxygenated blood to flow through muscles.

There are many different types of massage, and you may have to try several before you find one that suits you best. Some of the most popular include:

Deep Tissue Massage ➶ This is my favourite, though it can be quite painful. It is used to treat chronic muscular tension.

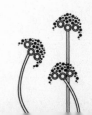

Neuromuscular Massage ᗡ Concentrates on a particular muscle and uses pressure on certain reflex points.

Esalen Massage ᗡ This is slow, rhythmic and relaxing.

Sports Massage ᗡ This is best done either immediately before or after exercising and consists of kneading and stretching muscles to increase flexibility.

Aromatherapy Massage ᗡ Uses essential oils and a combination of various strokes, depending on the particular therapist. I find it's worth shopping around until you find someone whose touch you're happy with.

I have a massage every week now and I treat it as an essential part of body maintenance. My therapist combines deep tissue sports massage with manual lymph drainage. Ronnie loves the massages I give him. He says it is because I know his body so well and with all the massages I have had I should know what I am doing!

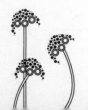

Exercise and Relaxation

Ayurveda

Ayurveda is the oldest documented body of holistic medical knowledge and it originated in India over 6,000 years ago. It uses plant oils and herbs to heal, but is far broader in reach than the purely medical, focusing on the flow of energy around us, and how the various factors in our environment affect our health or ill-health. It's about learning how to keep well rather than curing ills and – like yoga – it accepts the interconnectedness of mind, body and spirit and aims to balance all three.

I became fascinated by Ayurveda when I was in Arizona, staying at a wonderful spa called Miraval, where I was given an extraordinary massage during which oil was dripped slowly on to my third eye. Later, on tour in India, I had more wonderful Ayurvedic massages and treatments and fell in love with the oils they used. One night, in the heart of Mumbai, we went to a fabulous party at this mystical house, where I met the two great guys who run the company that produces the Kama Ayurveda products, using old Ayurvedic recipes. They got me hooked, and I was so inspired that I couldn't wait to get back to London to start making my own oils.

Ayurveda teaches moderation in all things, and the avoidance of excess. Not very rock 'n' roll, but there we go. One of the essential

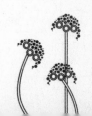

cornerstones of Ayurveda is the belief that the most important relationship is the one you have with yourself, and I think this is something I have really come to understand over the past five years.

Ayurveda shows a wise understanding of what happens when life gets out of balance – the kind of state I was in after touring unhealthily for so many years. The answer is to try and 'ground' yourself, to reconnect with what is important to you. The following visualisation technique is one of the ways that helps do that:

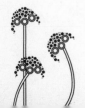 Think back to a time from your earlier life when you felt safe, happy and relaxed. I like to recall the moments when, as a very young child, I used to stand on a stool in my mum's kitchen helping her stir cake mixture, make fudge or roll pastry.

Feel how simple and pure the feeling is as you remember your younger self.

Hold this feeling and luxuriate in it, try to let it blot out your current feelings of unhappiness or unease.

Think about some ways in which you could simplify your life, or set aside some time to calm yourself – maybe something as simple as a bath full of fragrant oils (works for me) – and while you are doing that, reevaluate your priorities with the aim of focusing your energies on just a few things.

🐝 Find a trusted friend or mentor who might be able to advise you further. Ayurveda is big on advising people to find wise elders to guide them.

This act of looking inside yourself, trying to get in touch with the person you once were, is also a way of connecting with nature. It will help you to feel more grounded if you do this exercise whenever you feel overworked, under-appreciated or cut off from who you really are or want to be. Ayurveda is also big on the importance of cleansing your body, to make sure you eliminate waste products efficiently and regularly. Perhaps, with my history of colon catastrophe, this is why it appeals to me, knowing how my life turned around once I was eating a cleansing diet. It's all about flows of energy – if your intestines are obstructed with toxic stuff – known as '*ama*' in Ayurveda – then you'll feel dull, listless, even ill. If you become sick, it is nature's wake-up call to return to a healthier, more balanced existence. Remove the cause, and the effect will disappear.

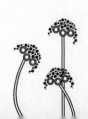

Your Face and Body

Ayurveda has some complex dietary rules, but they seem sensible and aren't too difficult to adapt to your own life and regime:

🐝 Eat only after you have digested your previous meals.

🌸 Leave at least two hours between your last meal and going to bed.

🐝 Make food for other people – the gift of food can be the best food of all.

🌸 Feed all five senses – take time to appreciate the smell, taste and sight of your food.

🐝 Drink only a little warm water during your meal.

🌸 Don't eat when you are not hungry, or when you are angry or depressed.

🐝 Do not exercise or work immediately after food.

🌸 Do not waste food.

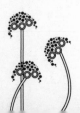

🐝 Say grace – particularly meaningful if you have grown and harvested your own vegetables.

✿ You're also supposed to eat quietly, without laughing or talking, but I find this one pretty near impossible.

REIKI

Reiki is not just another therapy; it is a special kind of healing. At the heart of reiki is the desire to make someone 'whole' again. I first discovered it at the health spa Champneys. As with many other complementary therapies, it starts with the aim of improving someone's health, but at the same time heals the mind and spirit too. The word reiki comes from the Japanese, and means 'universal life energy'. It refers to the life force as *ki*, the vital energy in all life that the yogis call *prana* and the Chinese call *chi*. I wonder why it is only in the western world we need this explained to us, when it is so much taken for granted in the east. I have felt this sense of calmness in my travels, especially in Japan.

The reiki practitioner, using certain hand positions on and over different parts of your body, channels this energy and uses it to release

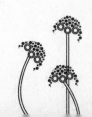

blocked energy, cleanse the body of toxins and re-balance it. The body's own self-healing powers are activated. A treatment usually lasts an hour, with each hand position being held for about three minutes. It is brilliant for stress, migraine, back pain, depression and other chronic conditions.

For practitioners of reiki, it is a spiritual path as well as a method of healing. There are five principles of reiki, which for me express fundamental truths about the way our lives could be improved:

ᎧᏓ

1 Just for today do not worry.

2 Just for today do not anger.

3 Honour your parents, teachers and elders.

4 Earn your living honestly.

5 Show gratitude for everything.

ᎧᏓ

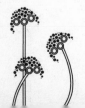

REFLEXOLOGY

My sister introduced me to reflexology in 1990. I used to hate people touching my feet, but she convinced me to try it and I was converted. In essence, it is foot massage and, as I have since found after a night of dancing, there is nothing nicer than going for reflexology the next day.

But there is far more to it than this. A reflexologist is someone who knows how to apply pressure to certain reflex points on the feet. According to eastern medicine, channels of energy run through the body, and there are points on our feet that correspond directly to parts of our body. Think acupuncture. A 'reflex' is the body's unconscious response to a stimulus, and when reflex points on the foot are activated they spark off a reaction in the particular organs and glands connected to the point. It follows that any part of your body that is not working properly can be helped by stimulating the relevant point.

If you think about it, we expect our feet to carry us through life but we treat them pretty badly – we squash them into tight shoes, overload them with weight, walk, jog and run on them. I'm one of the worse offenders – I used to love my spiky heels, I adore dancing and I enjoy running. But as I started to get more in touch

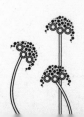

with the earth through yoga, where you stretch and wiggle your bare feet, I became much more aware of my feet. It sounds odd, but they are what connects us to the earth, they 'ground' us. If they are not treated well there is a danger we will feel lost, stressed or unhappy.

It's not a magic trick that will work all by itself. I believe we all have to take responsibility for our health, and that involves looking at all kinds of different approaches, including the ones I have discussed in this chapter. However, reflexology is certainly a very calming, comforting experience, and if that doesn't help with stress I don't know what would. A relaxed, balanced body is in the best shape to heal itself.

There's much more to all these therapies than I can tell you in this chapter. Indeed, I've been learning about them for some time now and I feel I've only scratched the surface myself. I am convinced, though, that the movement towards the acceptance of the gentle eastern disciplines of yoga, Ayurveda, massage, reflexology and reiki can only get stronger and that, increasingly, people will appreciate their ability to enhance our bodies' capacity to self-heal and will embrace their emphasis on the importance of nutrition as the foundation of good health.

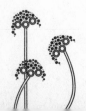

Exercise and Relaxation

Thank God I found an organic way of life. If I hadn't, I'd be in a terrible state by now. Touring is great fun, but can be incredibly stressful – flying all over the place, meeting loads of new people, eating different foods and drinking different water, partying, living in hotels . . . it all takes its toll. I am thankful I am stronger and healthier because of my clean diet and exercise regime, but also that I know how to detox my mind and body when I get back to my twin sanctuaries of my home and my family.

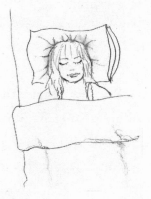

'Work like you don't need the money, dance like no one is watching, and love like you have never been hurt.'

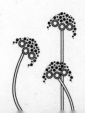

Your Face and Body

I prefer the stars and the moon
To a ceiling and a door

I prefer blue skies and countryside
To cities and buildings wide

I prefer fresh air and space
To any crowded place

I want pure stuff on my skin
More than any other thing

I want green and organic
To saturate our planet

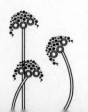

Exercise and Relaxation

I want silk and lace

To touch my face

I prefer natural and clean

Not chemical and fake

I want health and happiness

Not GMs and sprays

Let's change it now

In so many ways

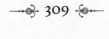

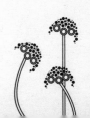

'**Eating organic** helps towards good health.'

Charlie R. Watts

Part 3

Creating a Greener Home

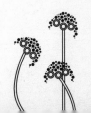

9

Cleaning the House

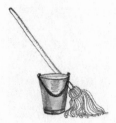

THERE'S MORE TO BEING ORGANIC than what you put into and on to your body and, as I delved more deeply in what it means to be green, I started thinking about the rest of my house. What was in the household cleaners? Were there chemicals lurking in the sheets on our bed? What should we be doing with all our rubbish? What about our energy use, our water, our furniture . . . ? Were we taking more from the planet than we were giving back? What sort of a world would my grandchildren be growing up in?

These thoughts bothered me, so I set about trying to do something about it. What I discovered was that it was far easier than I thought to make small changes. And even small changes can

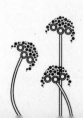

have a huge impact on the planet if we all make them. Here are a few ideas to get you started. See what you think – going green is not only simpler than you imagine, I truly believe it is the most important thing we can do.

'Josephine was always destined to be Deputy Mother Nature. She has immense capacity to see the beauty in natural things.'

Paul Karslake (Jo's brother)

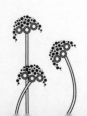

Cleaning the House

HOUSEHOLD PRODUCTS

I've already written about the dangers of our exposure to chemicals in the previous chapters, and some of the strongest ones we come into contact with are probably under your kitchen sink, in your laundry cupboard or under your stairs – wherever you stash your cleaning products. Conventional household cleaning products are strong and abrasive. They contain substances such as nonylphenol, chlorine, phosphates, petrochemicals and formaldehyde – and they do a great cleaning job. The only trouble is, they are toxic to humans and harmful to the environment.

Bleach ☠ Chlorine bleach (sodium hypochloride) is a key ingredient in lots of cleaning products. It is a lung and eye irritant and can create a toxic gas if you accidentally mix it with an acid-based cleaning product.

Petroleum-based Products ☠ These are made from coal tar, which is carcinogenic and – if poured down drains – ends up in the food chain.

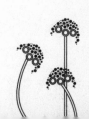

Phosphates ☠ These are mineral-based water softeners, which cause a rapid growth of algae in rivers. Although not used in many products these days, they are found in dishwasher detergent.

Triclosan ☠ An antibacterial found in toilet cleaners, deodorants and detergents which can cause infertility and organ failure. It is also toxic to aquatic life, and can end up in the food chain – a Swedish study of breastfeeding women found 60 per cent of them had triclosan in their breastmilk.

Volatile Organic Compounds ☠ Formaldehyde, toluene, styrene, xylenes, and trichloroethylene are all VOCs, which are manmade chemicals that include industrial solvents, fuel oxygenates and by-products of chlorination, such as chloroform. Many household products, including air fresheners, stain removers, cleaners, paint, paint strippers, varnish and glue, release volatile organic compounds into the air – and not just when the product is used, as the bottle or aerosol can release them while they are being stored. Not only do the fumes cause breathing difficulties, studies have also linked long-term exposure to cancer, birth defects and disruption of the hormones.

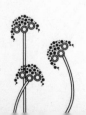

Cleaning the House

Lots of people have switched to gentler alternatives – products such as Ecover or Enviroclean – particularly now they are more widely available. They are not organic, but they are environmentally friendly. They use plant-based perfumes, are kinder to your skin, don't bubble up too much and don't leave unnecessary chemicals behind on your dishes, floors or surfaces. The ingredients used cause minimum harm to aquatic life and the products have been developed without animal testing. The bottles are biodegradable and can also be refilled. The laundry products do not use optical brightening agents (chemicals that reflect light to make your whites look whiter) as these have been found to be harmful to skin.

AIR FRESHENERS

Manufacturers don't need to list the chemicals in these products but they can include formaldehyde, phthalates and artificial fragrances. Rather than improving your air, these products simply add more chemicals to it. I particularly hate plug-in air fresheners which expose us to a continuous release of chemicals from the fragrance. The best way to get rid of a bad smell is to open the window, and clean the source of it.

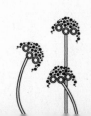

If you want your house or a room to smell nice, why not use a scented candle? It should be natural with organic ingredients and oils. Candles made from paraffin wax (a petrochemical derivative) can release soot, benzene and other VOCs as well as the chemicals making up the fragrance when they burn.

A few drops of your favourite essential oil on a burner will fragrance a room, or you can buy organic room sprays from the Organic Pharmacy (see page 363 for contact details).

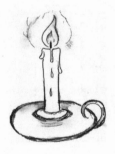

REAL ALTERNATIVES

When I was first setting up home with Ronnie, my mum passed on all sorts of cleaning tips that really work. Don't think of them as old fashioned, think of them as retro. Here are some of my mum's, with

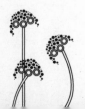

extras I have discovered for myself – they'll mean you won't have to reach for the bleach, and you'll feel like a worthy wartime mum wearing a pinny.

WHITE VINEGAR

This is top of my list – and I always have some to hand – as it can be used for a hundred and one little cleaning jobs around the house. It is brilliant for descaling kettles (boil with half vinegar, half water) and taps and showerheads (fix a bag full of vinegar over the showerhead or tap and leave overnight). To clean windows and mirrors, polish with vinegar and newspaper. Or use on a soft cloth for stainless-steel surfaces. Leave half a pint in the loo overnight; add it to dishwasher detergent for shinier glasses; or add it neat and run the dishwasher through a cycle to clean it. Vinegar and water left overnight in a burned saucepan will make it easier to clean in the morning. Get into the habit of adding a splash of it to your washing-up water for sparkling dishes. And wipe mouldy shower curtains with vinegar before washing.

BICARBONATE
OF SODA

If you have a blocked drain, pour a tablespoon of bicarbonate of soda down the drain, followed by a cup of white vinegar, then flush it with boiling water. You may have to repeat a few times. This should dissolve grease and ease blockages (a plunger may help too).

Sprinkle on grimy pans, ovens or baths to lift the dirt more easily.

A solution of warm water and bicarbonate of soda (1 tbs bicarb to half a pint of water) will clean a musty Thermos and remove coffee and tea stains from plastic cups and dishes.

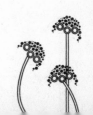

BICARBONATE OF SODA (CONT.)	*It's also a good alternative to your harsh toilet cleaner: sprinkle in the bowl, add some white vinegar and scrub vigorously – don't expect to be able to leave it to do the work for you.*
	You can also use it as a carpet cleaner: sprinkle liberally on your carpet and vacuum off after half an hour.
VANILLA	*A few drops of vanilla extract on a cotton wool ball will scent a fridge or drawer.*
LEMON	*Squeeze a little juice on stains on clothes, leave to dry, then wash out. White cotton socks past their best can be freshened up by boiling them up with a slice of lemon.*
	Rub lemon juice on to your hands to remove food smells.
	Dip a lemon into salt and rub into your wooden chopping board to clean it. Also works well on silver.
ORANGE PEEL	*Place in a warm oven to help get rid of cooking smells.*
CHARCOAL	*Helps eliminate smells in the fridge or shoe cupboard.*
ESSENTIAL OILS	*Burn citronella, lavender or tea tree to get rid of unpleasant smells. The latter is particularly good in the lavatory bowl as it is a mild disinfectant.*
SALT	*Sprinkle liberally over dirty ovens and scrub like mad. (Though not in self-cleaning ovens.) Put a sheet of aluminium foil on the bottom of your oven to catch drips and spills and cleaning will be automatically easier.*

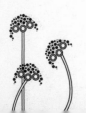

Cleaning the House

HERBS   *Chuck a handful into your bin to keep it sweet smelling, and use bay leaves, lavender or rosemary in your drawers to keep moths away.*

TEA   *Leave cold tea in a fish pan for ten minutes before washing it to reduce fishy smells*

MUSTARD   *A tablespoon of mustard powder in a smelly flower vase filled half with water will both clean and freshen the glass.*

WHITE WINE   *If you have any left over use it to clean glass shower doors.*

TOOTHPASTE   *Has a surprising number of uses — it's good for buffing up tarnished silver, cleaning the toes of trainers or football boots and even removing scratches on glassware.*

BEESWAX   *Much better for polishing furniture than the sprays. Even without ozone layer destroying CFCs they still contain unpleasant chemicals which can trigger asthma.*

It would also be a good idea to replace your aluminium and nonstick pans with stainless-steel ones, since aluminium and perfluorinated compounds are linked with cancer. It's also advisable to avoid phthalates, which are found in PVC products such as cling film, plastic utensils and baby beakers, as we just don't know enough about what the long-term effects of using them might be.

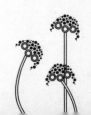

10

A Greener Home

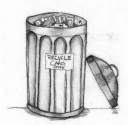

TEXTILES

In the light of what I was discovering about farming practices, hidden ingredients and fair trade, I started to look into organic textiles too. This may not be the easiest thing for everyone to change, but I'd like to get you thinking about why you should switch to organic clothes and bedding.

Cotton is used for a huge range of products and is one of the most widely traded substances on earth. It therefore has a massive impact on the earth's air, water and soil – as well as on the health of the people

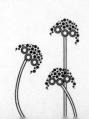

living in cotton-growing countries. In 1995, US farmers sprayed nearly 150 g of chemical fertilisers and pesticides for every 450 g of cotton harvested. To put this in context, it takes 450 g of cotton to make one T-shirt. After seven years of growing GM cotton, farmers in China have had to use over 400 per cent more pesticides to kill new 'secondary' pests. Around a quarter of the world's insecticides are used to grow cotton and at least 8,000 chemicals are used to turn raw material into clothes, towels, bedding and other items that we buy.

So, if you switch to buying organic textiles you will encourage more farmers to adopt organic and fair trade practices, with all the other attendant benefits of biodiversity and lower energy consumption that I have explained elsewhere. Most of the new clothes I buy are either organic, fair trade or vintage (even Ronnie's boxer shorts are organic). Habitat has started selling organic cotton towels, and many big clothing retailers are moving towards sourcing some of their cotton organically. This is great news, and I hope more big names will follow. Meanwhile, you'll find the internet is a great source of information about companies selling organic textiles – see the back of the book for some websites to get you started.

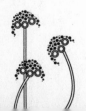

Reasons to Buy Organic Fibres

🐝 Conventional bedding is doused in chemicals, including boric acid — which is also used as rat poison — to increase its fire-retardant qualities.

🌸 Synthetic dye uses up a great deal of energy and produces lots of toxic waste. Natural colours are less polluting.

🐝 By choosing chemical-free fabrics you will reduce the chemical allergens in the environment, many of which are associated with an increased rate of developmental and behavioural problems in children.

🌸 Organic fabrics can be composted safely.

🐝 By buying organic fabrics you will be supporting fair trade practices and biodiversity.

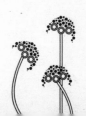

I want to briefly mention organic tampons. We consumers demand ever smaller and ever more absorbent tampons, which has led to the original cotton tampons being (if you'll pardon the pun) tampered with. They now contain synthetic materials such as viscose, rayon and plastic. Some also contain perfume and bleach, and – unless marked – the cotton they are made from is non organic and therefore has been sprayed with pesticides. These can all cause irritation to our most sensitive areas. More than that, there is a risk of toxic shock syndrome, which does still affect a very small number of people a year. It is unheard of in those who use organic cotton tampons. Look for brands such as Natracare – I've seen them next to the regular ones in my local supermarket.

FURNITURE

I've had most of my furniture for years, but there are some things to consider when buying new stuff. Consider how the piece was made, what it was made of, who made it, what kinds of materials it includes. Be aware, for example, of the harm done to the environment by non-sustainable woods, and the toxic chemicals in some synthetic furniture.

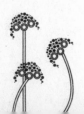

'Conventional cotton uses 24 per cent of all insecticides used each year; making products from organic cotton makes a huge difference to farmers, to consumers, and to the earth. Jo clearly understands this and has been a positive influence on us for many years. The more people she can reach with her message, and the more we can draw from her experiences, the better off the planet – and all of its inhabitants! – will be.'

William and Gabriela Lana,
founders Greenfibres

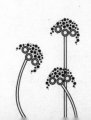

🐝 Try your local recycling centre, second-hand shop or auction house before rushing out to a shop. There are plenty of websites to help you.

❀ If you do have to buy new, try and find furniture that is made from reclaimed wood, is certified by a body such as the Forest Stewardship Council or SmartWood. I know that B&Q and The Pier do have some furniture made from sustainable wood.

🐝 Failing that, ask if the wood comes from well-managed forests and if the company has a 'closed loop' policy where they avoid the unnecessary harvesting of trees and disposal of wood into landfill sites.

❀ Look for furniture that is made without harmful adhesives, formaldehydes or VOCs (see page 316). These can trigger asthma and aggravate chest complaints and allergies.

🐝 Look for furniture made from recycled plastic.

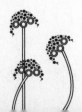

A Greener Home

DIY

Looking after a house is a bit like painting the Forth Bridge. You think you've finally finished and then you realise the room you started with looks scruffy and needs a facelift. When you're decorating, try to use natural materials and ask yourself whether you really need something new or whether you can find anything recycled or sustainable. There are loads of green and environmentally friendly products and approaches out there. Here are a few:

🐝 Go to architectural salvage sites.

🌸 Buy organic paint and products without petrochemicals.

🐝 Recycle paint you no longer need (see page 378 for information).

🌸 Find out if you are eligible for a grant to install an energy-saving device such as a solar panel, wind turbine, etc.

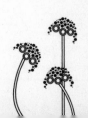

Creating a Greener Home

YOUR ENERGY CONSUMPTION

A third of all carbon emissions in the UK come from burning fossil fuels to generate electricity. An average home in this country produces around 5.6 tonnes of CO_2 per year – from heating, lighting and running electrical appliances. I have a dream that one day all households will generate their electricity at home, using wind, solar and heat energy. It's a long way off, I fear, and the government would need to invest so much in panels and turbines for public buildings that the costs would fall for the rest of us. Meanwhile, there are other things you can do. Use less energy, for a start. Clean your windows (with vinegar, remember) and let more natural light in. Switch off (low-energy) lights after leaving a room – I'm always shocked at how few people do this. Don't leave the TV on standby. When buying new white goods, check their energy efficiency. Simple actions can make a difference: lag your water tank, or insulate your loft – which in itself would save just under half a tonne of CO_2 a year – and investigate the possibility of solar panels. Change to a green energy supplier (I use Ecotricity, a company that invests in new sources of renewable energy). I'm also excited by the idea of having a wind turbine at home to provide some of our power.

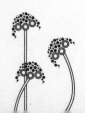

A Greener Home

Rub Out Your Carbon Footprint

The other thing Ronnie and I did was to have our home carbon-neutralised (see page 380 for details on who to contact to do this). This is a simple but brilliant idea whereby the amount of carbon dioxide generated by you and your family in a year is calculated, and in compensation you invest in reforestation and renewable energy projects. With all the flying we do – did you know that one single short-haul flight produces about the same amount of the global warming gas as three months' worth of driving a 1.4 litre car? – we ended up planting thousands of trees.

Save Water

The drought last summer brought it all home to us just how much water we are wasting, whether we are brushing our teeth, showering, washing vegetables, hosing down the car or flushing the loo. Get a water butt, buy a hippo for the lavatory cistern (shockingly, flushing accounts for more than a third of our domestic water use); make sure your washing machine is full when you use it or use short cycles; use a washing-up bowl rather than the whole sink. I'm fanatical about

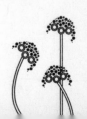

rinsing bubbles off my plates, but I use a second bowl of clean water to rinse dishes in rather than holding them under a running tap. Once you've finished with it, chuck the water on the garden – even if it's been raining.

RECYCLE

I have to admit that my passion for recycling started with shopping. Everywhere I go I frequent flea markets and vintage clothing stores, and some of my favourite possessions are those which many previous owners have enjoyed. My collection of antique French scent bottles, for example, provided the inspiration for my own products, and my attic is full of gorgeous clothes dating back some thirty years. The other night I was looking for something to wear to our annual Woodfest party, and I remembered a black sequin dress I hadn't worn for years. It was the perfect choice!

I have mentioned my friend Lorraine in the book a couple of times. She has a fabulous boutique in New York called Geminola. Lorraine works with beautiful vintage fabrics, none of which date any earlier than the 1950s, so this is another great example of how we can all recycle and also have an exquisite wardrobe.

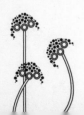

A Greener Home

On the household front, I recycle everything – glass, plastics, paper and cans. Greener World even awarded us a certificate for the most bottles recycled in a year. Think before you throw anything away. On average, each household in the UK throws away 1 tonne of rubbish a year. It's too easy just to consign it to the bin or skip – don't do it. Check the internet for the hundreds of sites that will take away your unwanted goods from old mobile phones to printers to children's toys; or take them to car boot sales and charity shops.

When you're shopping, avoid heavily packaged goods, and try to select only those with biodegradable or recyclable packaging. Even better, buy 'loose' food. Take your own shopping bag (each person in the UK uses an average of 134 plastic bags each year and only a small number are biodegradable).

Contact the Mail Preference Service (0845 703 4599 or via the website *www.mpsonline.org.uk*) and get your name taken off the junk mail list, and try putting a polite notice on your front door asking that no junk mail be put through your letterbox. This will help reduce waste.

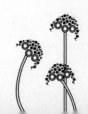

A Final Word

My journey into a more natural way of living began when I fell ill.
You may already have taken some steps on your own journey, or
you may only just have begun thinking about making some changes
to the way you eat, shop and live. Whoever you are, wherever you
live, whatever your lifestyle and politics, I hope that you have found
something in this book to inspire you. Let's keep ourselves, and the
planet, naturally gorgeous.

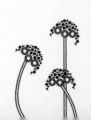

A Final Word

I savour the moment when my work is done

and I find somewhere to sit and be the only one

I savour the moment with the wind in my hair

at that moment in time I love that I'm there

I savour the moment I wish it would last

but it's there then it's gone and is now in the past

᷍᷍᷍

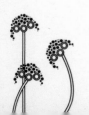

A Final Word

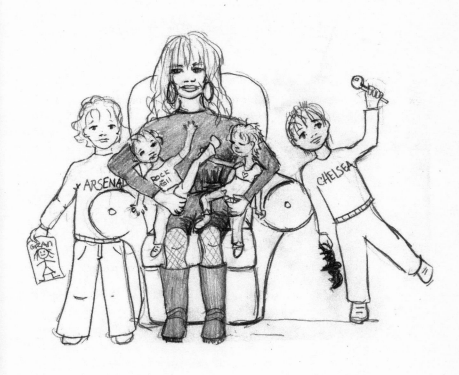

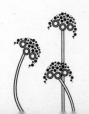

Information on Organics

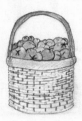

There are relatively few books on living organically, so if you're interested in finding out more about organic and green issues, the internet is probably the best place to start. The following are some of the most helpful organisations and websites.

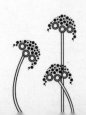

Information on Organics

The Soil Association

Bristol House, 40–56 Victoria Street, Bristol BS1 6BY
Tel: 0117 314 5000
Soil Association Scotland, 18 Liberton Brae, Tower Mains,
Edinburgh EH16 6AE
Tel: 0131 666 2474

A charitable organisation that promotes and certifies organic food and farming and sustainable forestry. They have a fantastic website that offers lots of information on organic issues and is therefore a good place to start. You can register on the site (for free) with *whyorganic.org*, which gives you access to their directory of organic producers and services in Britain and to their food club.
www.soilassociation.org

Pesticide Action Network

Development House, 56–64 Leonard Street,
London EC2A 4JX
Tel: 020 7065 0905

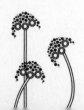

Information on Organics

An international non-profit organisation that works to promote healthy food, agriculture and an environment which will provide food and meet public health needs without dependence on toxic chemicals, and without harm to food producers and agricultural workers. Although it provides other information as well, their website is particularly good on pesticides in food and gardening tips. *www.pan-uk.org*

ᴔᴂ

Women's Environmental Network

PO Box 30626, London E1 1TZ
Tel: 020 7481 9004

A charity that campaigns on environmental and health issues from a female perspective, with local groups around Britain. *www.wen.org.uk*

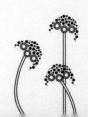

Chemicalfree.co.uk

Chemical Free, 56 Gaping Lane,
Hitchin, Herts SG5 2JE

If you are affected by multiple chemical sensitivity or multiple food intolerance then this website will help with information and support.
www.chemicalfree.co.uk

෮෮

Friends of the Earth

26–28 Underwood Street,
London NI 7JQ
Tel: 020 7490 1555

An international organisation that campaigns on environmental issues.
www.foe.co.uk

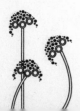

The World Wildlife Fund

WWF-UK, Panda House, Weyside Park, Godalming, Surrey GU7 1XR
Tel: 01483 426333 (for supporters and information)

An international body that works to conserve endangered species, to protect threatened habitats and address global threats – including the threat to us all of hazardous chemicals. Click on to *www.wwf.org.uk/ chemicals/indecent_exposure.asp* to do an online test to assess your own exposure to toxic chemicals.
www.wwf.org.uk

66

Greenpeace

Canonbury Villas, London N1 2PN
Tel: 020 7865 8100

An international non-profit organisation that focuses on threats to the planet's biodiversity and ecology. The website contains a lot of useful information about the chemicals in our homes – for more information log on to *www.greenpeace.org.uk/Products/Toxics/chemicalhouse.cfm*.
www.greenpeace.org.uk

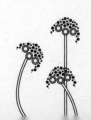

Tusk Trust
5 Townbridge House, High Street,
Gillingham, Dorset SP8 4AA
Tel: 01747 831 005

This organisation has over fifteen years experience initiating and funding conservation and community development programmes right across Africa.
www.tusk.org

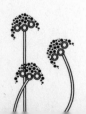

Where to Buy
Organic Products

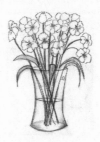

Again, there's lots of information on the internet – these websites are a good place to start if you're trying to source organic products.

About Organics ↝ An online consumer guide that provides information on leading an achievable healthy and organic

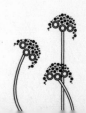

lifestyle, with advice and links to retailers throughout the UK and Eire. Includes lists of local organic retailers, box schemes, restaurants, producers, holidays and much more.
www.aboutorganics.co.uk

Guide Me Green ᛞ A website that promotes green companies and brands and provides both an ethical directory and a green directory.
www.guidemegreen.com

Hippy Shopper ᛞ A fun newsblog devoted to greener and more ethical shopping. Whether you want organic knickers, eco-friendly clothing or just a link to your nearest farmers' market, it's all here.
www.hippyshopper.com

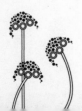

Where to Buy Organic Products

Spirit of Nature ✲ Sells more than 600 natural and environmentally friendly products, many organic – includes organic clothing and cosmetics, eco-friendly household products and nappies and toys.
www.spiritofnature.co.uk

ORGANIC SHOPS

As Nature Intended

Currently this company has two stores in London:

🐝 17–21 High Street, Ealing, London W5 5DB
✿ 201 Chiswick High Road, London W4 2DR
www.asnatureintended.uk.com

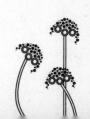

Bumblebee

Sells vegetarian, organic and wholefoods and eco-friendly household products. They also offer a box delivery scheme to some north London postcodes, and a mail order service for England and Wales. To order you can use their website, call 020 7607 1935 or email *info@bumblebee.co.uk*

30 Brecknock Road, London, N7 0DD
www.bumblebee.co.uk

ଚ୍ଚ

Fresh and Wild

Britain's largest organic and natural food retailer, with stores in London and Bristol, which recently joined with the American company Whole Foods Market.

 Camden Town, 49 Parkway, London NW1 7PN
 Clapham Junction, 305–311 Lavender Hill, London SW11 1LN
 Clifton, Bristol, 85 Queen's Road, Bristol BS8 1QS
 Notting Hill, 208–212 Westbourne Grove, London W11 2RH

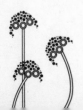

Where to Buy Organic Products

🐝 Soho, 69–75 Brewer Street, London WIF 9US

🌸 Stoke Newington, 32–40 Stoke Newington Church Street,
   London N16 0LU

www.freshandwild.com

☙❧

Planet Organic

An organic supermarket with three branches in London.

🐝 25 Effie Road, Fulham, London SW6 1EL

🌸 42 Westbourne Grove, London W2 5SH

🐝 22 Torrington Place, London WC1 7JE

They also have a home delivery service. To order, email *deliveries@
planetorganic.com*

www.planetorganic.com

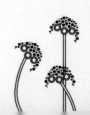

OTHER SOURCES OF ORGANIC FOOD

Organicfood.co.uk

For general information you might want look at this internet magazine. It includes a listing of box schemes and shops selling organic produce in your local area.
www.organicfood.co.uk

☯

Farmers Markets

A great place to browse and find wonderful new products. Not everything is organic, but it will all be locally produced and fresh from the farm. Check *www.farmersmarkets.net*, which lists the markets certified by FARMA (the National Farmers' Retail and Markets Association) who inspect them to make sure that the food is local and that the producer or someone involved in the production of the food will be on hand to give customers information. There's also a list of certified and uncertified markets at the back of *Organic Life* magazine.

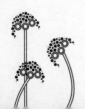

Box Schemes

These are a great way of getting fresh organic produce delivered from the farm to your door. There are too many schemes across the country for me to list them all here. The Soil Association website and Organicfood.co.uk have a listing, as does *Organic Life* magazine. It's worth looking at suppliers' websites to see what selections they offer, and which you prefer. Delivery times may vary from supplier to supplier also.

Abel & Cole

16 Waterside Way, Plough Lane, Wimbledon SW17 0HB
Tel: 08452 626262 / 020 8944 3780

Deliver fresh organic fruit and vegetables and meat, sustainably sourced fish and other ethically produced foods. They offer the full range across London and parts of the Home Counties and towns in south and west England. They also offer a smaller range that covers most of the rest of the country.
www.abel-cole.co.uk

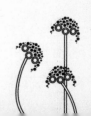

Where to Buy Organic Products

Farmaround

The Old Bakery, Mercury Road, Richmond, North Yorkshire
DL10 4TQ

Supply organic vegetables and fruit boxes to the London area and,
via *www.farmaroundnorth.co.uk*, North Yorkshire and the north east of
England. Order via the website.
www.farmaround.co.uk

☙❧

Riverford

Riverford Organic Vegetables Limited, Wash Barn, Buckfastleigh,
Devon TQ11 0LD
Tel: 01803 762720

Based at Riverford Farm in Devon, this organic box scheme is
available through most of southern England and, via River Nene
Organic Vegetables, the eastern counties. As well as the basic boxes
of vegetables you can add a range of organic produce, from eggs and
dairy to jam and wine. You can order via the website.
www.riverford.co.uk

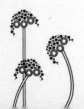

Mail Order

You can also source organic food by mail order. Again, there are lots of suppliers but these are a couple of the best known.

Graig Farm Organics

Dolau, Llandrindod Wells, Powys LD1 5TL
Tel: 01597 851655

An award-winning organic mail order service — organic vegetable boxes, meat and dairy, organic and sustainable farmed fish, baked goods, wine and beer, plus products such as cosmetics and herbal remedies.
www.graigfarm.co.uk

Daylesford Organic

near Kingham, Gloucestershire GL56 0YG
Tel: 0800 0831233

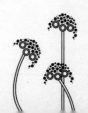

Supply organic vegetables, fruit and herbs, bread, meat, groceries and wine, plus household products and paint. You can also visit the farm shop, or order online at *mailorder@daylesfordorganic.com* *www.daylesfordorganic.com*

ᘓᘐ

Swaddles Farm

Swaddles Organic, The Laurels, Poets Way, Newham, Northamptonshire NN11 3HQ
Tel: 0845 456 1768

Organic butchers who, in addition to their award-winning meat, sell fruit, vegetables and herbs on line. You can pick up your order from the farm, or they have a weekly delivery in their own refrigerated vans to London and parts of Surrey and Middlesex, and deliver by overnight carrier in other parts of the UK. You can shop online and order by email *orders@swaddles.co.uk*.
www.swaddles.co.uk

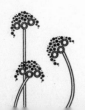

Where to Buy Organic Products

Vintage Roots

Farley Farms, Bridge Farm, Reading Road, Arborfield, Berkshire
RG2 9HT
Tel: 0800 9804992

Suppliers of organic and diodynamic wines, beer and spirits from around the world. You can request a mail-order catalogue via their website or order online.
www.vintageroots.co.uk

ORGANIC BREAD

One of my passions, so I hope you will search out your local organic baker. Check out *www.danlepard.com* for a list of local artisan bakeries. Many organic box delivery schemes will offer bread as well. If you're in Hastings, you should pop into my friend Jo's bakery: Judges Bakery, 51 High Street, Hastings Old Town TN34 3EN.

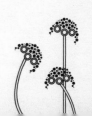

The Village Bakery

Melmerby, Penrith, Cumbria CA10 1HE

Tel: 01768 881811

Organic artisan bread, cakes and biscuits from this pioneering organic bakery are available from some supermarkets and health food shops around the country but they also have an online mail order service. You can also buy from their shop at Melmerby.

www.village-bakery.com

ETHICAL EATING

Happy Cow

This website gives a guide to vegetarian restaurants and health food shops around the world.

www.happycow.net

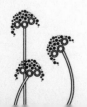

Where to Buy Organic Products

Eat the Seasons

This site gives comprehensive advice on what food is in season each month – with information on nutritional value, what to look for when buying the food and how to cook it. It has links to recipes if you are in need of inspiration.

www.eattheseasons.co.uk

Big Barn

Type in your postcode and you will be supplied with a list of locally produced food. This is a great way to help with the food miles debate and supports local businesses. The site also contains recipes.

www.bigbarn.co.uk

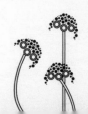

GARDENING

Garden Organic

The website of the Henry Doubleday Research Institute, a charity for organic growing, is full of useful information about organic gardening, including how to grow organic food and make compost and leafmould.

www.gardenorganic.org.uk

❧

The Organic Gardening Catalogue

The official catalogue of Garden Organic. A great source of organic seeds for vegetables – both heritage and modern varieties – fruit plants, herbs, flowers, green manures, organic composts and fertilisers, and biological pest controls. You can browse online or order a catalogue to be posted to you.

www.organiccatalog.com

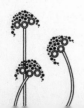

Tamar Organics

Another online gardening catalogue with over 400 varieties of organic seeds.

www.tamarorganics.co.uk

COSMETIC AND BEAUTY PRODUCTS

I'm glad to say it's fairly easy to buy organic beauty products these days – not just from health shops but also from department stores and, of course, over the internet. There are also natural products available which avoid those nasty chemicals. There are lots of lovely brands – too many, in fact, to mention them all – but here are some of the ones I like and which you should be able to get hold of without much difficulty.

Dr Hauschka

A German line of organic skincare and make-up (certified by Germany's regulatory body BDIH) based on plant ingredients grown and harvested biodynamically. It is available from John Lewis

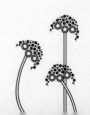

and Fenwicks department stores and health shops, as well as online.
www.drhauschka.co.uk

☙❧

Green People

A wide range of natural and organic beauty products – including toothpaste, sunscreen, shampoos and lipstick. Their products are available from health shops; you can also order online or by mail order, telephone: 01403 740 350.
www.greenpeople.co.uk

☙❧

Jurlique

An Australian brand that uses plants and herbs grown organically on their own farms. The range is also ph balanced and hypoallergenic. It is available from House of Fraser stores, but you can also order online or by telephone on 0870 770 0980.
www.jurlique.co.uk or *www.jurlique.com.au*

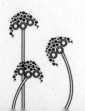

Kama Ayurveda

Authentica ayurveda products that are completely natural, using ingredients from organically grown plants and herbs.
www.kamaayurveda.com

☙❧

Lavera

Another German brand of organic and natural bodycare products for men, women and children. They also have a make-up range formulated for sensitive skin.
www.lavera.co.uk

☙❧

Liz Earle

22 Union Street, Ryde, Isle of Wight

A natural skincare range using organically grown ingredients or those sustainably harvested from the wild wherever possible. They

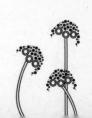

have a shop on the Isle of Wight (where the company is based) or you can order online.
www.lizearle.com

⊗⊗

Neal's Yard

Natural beauty products for women, men and babies. Organic ingredients are used wherever possible and some of their products are certified by the Soil Association. They have shops around the country – where you can also get advice on homeopathic and herbal remedies – and their products are also available in health shops and department stores including Harrods, Liberty, John Lewis, Fenwicks and Jenners. Their products are available online, or for mail order call 0845 262 3145.
www.nealsyardremedies.com

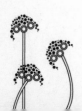

The Organic Pharmacy

396 Kings Road, London SW10 0LN
169 Kensington High Street, London W8 6SH

Specialises in herbs, homeopathy and a wide range of organic skincare – body and face products, sun cream, shampoos, mother and baby products. In addition to the two London stores they have an online ordering service.
www.theorganicpharmacy.com

REN

A green skincare collection that is free from all nasty chemicals and uses the latest discoveries in bioactive technology to promise great results. It is available from Liberty, John Lewis, House of Fraser and Selfridges and you can also order online or by phone on 0845 22 55 600.
www.renskincare.com

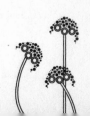

Spiezia Organics

A lovely range of beauty products for women, men and babies certified by the Soil Association. Products are available at Harvey Nichols and can be ordered online or by telephone on 0870 850 8851.

www.spieziaorganics.com

Weleda

Swiss organic beauty products, available from health stores, some larger branches of Sainsbury's, and online. You can also email for skincare advice via the website.

www.weleda.co.uk

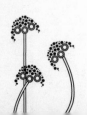

Jo Wood Organics

Jo Wood Organics is an ultra-luxurious collection of organic bath and skincare products. The entire collection is manufactured in Devon, England, from only the highest grade organic essential oils, active plant extracts and essential essences harvested from the best growing areas around the world. The products contain no animal ingredients; no artificial colours or fragrances; no genetically modified ingredients; no petroleum derivatives; no mineral oils; no sodium laureth sulphates; no parabens or phthalates; no chemically derived active ingredients and no water. Instead, they contain Sicilian organic orange juice ultra-filtered to the point where it becomes what is known as vegetal water, which has similar properties to water, but also has additional health-giving benefits.

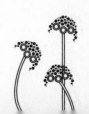

Jo Wood Organics comprises five luxurious body products in two distinct signature fragrances, Amka and Usiku. Each product has been carefully formulated to soothe, nourish and restore the skin to its natural radiance whilst helping to counteract the effects of ageing. The two fragrances have been structured in delicate layers from the finest organic essential oils, with cedarwood from Morocco; cardamom, ginger and cloves from the Far East; and bergamot and rosemary picked on the wild coasts of the Mediterranean.

Amka – meaning 'to wake' in Swahili – has a romantic heart of Iranian rose otto and Egyptian jasmine with bright, fresh top notes of neroli and bergamot; it is an energetic and spontaneous fragrance. Green mandarin and sweet orange add a fresh, vibrant layer above a soft and spicy base of cedarwood.

Usiku – meaning 'night' in Swahili – is warm and sensual with a fresh, vibrant edge; its earthy and sophisticated nature makes it suitable for both

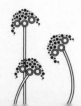

men and women. With top notes of rosemary and pine needle, it has a spicy hint of cardamom and hot ginger; a complex heart of coriander, clove and clary sage; and an aromatic, woody base of Moroccan cedarwood, patchouli and vetiver.

All organic ingredients are from accredited and audited sources and Jo Wood Organics is committed to working with suppliers to boost the production of organic crops. Not only have the products been tested on Jo's family and friends, but they also comply with all relevant European and FDA safety regulations.

'Jo Wood Organics are my favourite, I adore them. They smell delicious and make your wrinkles disappear.'

Jerry Hall

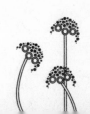

The Collection

Sold individually or in luxury gift sets, the Jo Wood Organics collection is available from Beyond Beauty at Harvey Nichols UK stores and worldwide through Selfridges, Neiman Marcus (selected stores), Bergdorf Goodman and selected independent stockists – see the website for a complete listing. You can also order from the website *www.jowoodorganics.com* or via mail order on +44(0)845 607 6614.

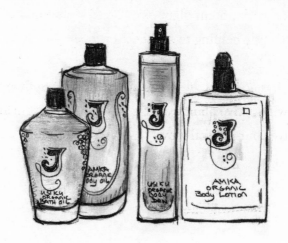

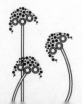

Amka Organic Bath Oil ↬ A reviving bath oil packed full of the energy of nature to enliven the body and brighten the spirits.

Usiku Organic Bath Oil ↬ A sensual and soothing bath oil to warm the heart and lift the spirits.

Amka Organic Body Lotion ↬ A deeply moisturising and firming lotion with potent plant seed oils to bring dull skin back to life.

Usiku Organic Body Lotion ↬ A smoothing, firming lotion with potent plant extracts to plump up the skin while helping to soothe and repair.

Amka Organic Body Oil ↬ A rich, regenerating body oil with active plant extracts to repair your skin and revive your natural glow.

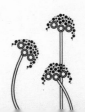

Usiku Organic Body Oil ᐧᕋ A rich, nourishing body oil with active plant extracts to smooth the skin and boost the immune system.

Usiku Organic Body Soap ᐧᕋ A rich, velvety, nourishing soap combining the healing properties of Mexican honey with softening extracts of oatmeal.

Amka Organic Body Dew ᐧᕋ A fine spray of active plant extracts and flower essences to revive body and soul.

Usiku Organic Body Dew ᐧᕋ A fine sensuous spray that energises the body and treats the skin with the woody Usiku aroma.

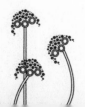

ESSENTIAL OILS

Essential oils are widely available in health shops and department stores but they may not always be organic. You can source them online from these companies:

Natural by Nature Oils Ltd

An award winning company using natural and organic essential oils and aromatherapy products. They are available from health food stores throughout the UK or by mail order, telephone 01582 840848.

www. naturalbynature.co.uk

৪৫৫

Neal's Yard

A wide range of organic essential oils which can be ordered online – see above for details.

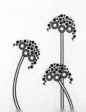

Quinessence Aromatherapy

Supply a wide range of organic essential oils that can be ordered online.

www.quinessence.com

Tisserand

Their range includes organic and wild-crafted oils, and their website says they are happy to give free advice for general enquiries if you call 01273 325666 or email *info@tisserand.com*. You can also order online.

www.tisserand.com

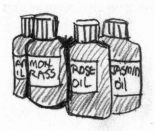

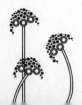

A Greener Home

Household Products

In addition to those listed below, also look for products from Daylesford Organic (see page 353). If you're shopping in Waitrose or John Lewis you'll find the Method range, an eco-friendly brand of natural cleaners from America, while Marks & Spencer has its Naturally Inspired range.

Ecover
This is probably the most widely available brand of eco-friendly household products, with at least some of the range carried by most major supermarkets and health food stores. Their website has information on stockists, and also on how to order online.
www.ecover.com

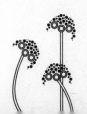

Sonett

Eco-friendly cleaning products using biodynamic and organic ingredients. Available from Green Fibres (see below).

www.sonett.co.uk

TEXTILES

Ecocentric

Sells fair trade and recyled products, including a cosmetics bag made from juice cartons, and beautiful glass.

www.ecocentric.co.uk

Green Fibres

Suppliers of organic textiles, including clothing, bedding and towels, as well as skincare and homeware products. Also available from Spirit of Nature (see page 347).

www.greenfibres.com

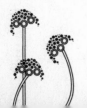

Hug.co.uk

Supply Fairtrade and organic cotton clothes.
www.hug.co.uk

DIY

Auro

Environmentally friendly paints and wood finishes. Check out the
website for a list of stockists or call 01452 772020.
www.auro.co.uk

Daylesford Organic

Also supplies environmentally friendly paint – see page 353 for
contact details.

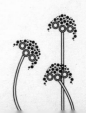

ECOS Organic Paints

Environmentally friendly paint with a range of 108 colours plus a colour matching service. You can order a brochure from the website or by calling 01795 418 218.

www.ecospaints.com

ᘒᘒ

The Good Wood Guide

Information on making the best choice when buying or using wood for your next DIY, self-build or construction project.

www.goodwoodguide.com

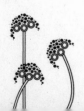

Going Green

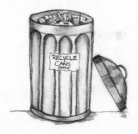

The Centre for Alternative Technology
Machynlleth, Powys SY20 9AZ
Tel: 01654 705950

Aims to inspire, inform and enable people to live more sustainably.
They offer a free information service on sustainable living: everything
from changing your light bulbs to building a new house. They will help
you reduce your environmental impact, lower your carbon footprint

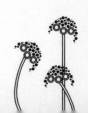

and reduce your energy bills. As well as the advice on the website, they will answer specific queries by email, post or telephone.
www.cat.org.uk

RECYCLING

Community Repaint
Will distribute your old usable paint to those who cannot afford it. Check out the website for your nearest scheme or contact Mark Gregory on 0113 200 3951, or email *mark.gregory@resourcefutures.co.uk*.
www.communityrepaint.org.uk

৪৫

Forever Green
Ecological architects who offer eco building design.
www.forevergreen.org.uk

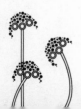

Geminola

41 Perry Street, New York, NY 10014

A lovely boutique with clothes made from vintage fabrics.
Tel: (001) 212 675 1994
www.geminola.com

Greener World

A company that collects products to recycle, from both businesses and households.
www.greenerworld.com

Reuze.co.uk

A website that supplies information on how, what and where you can recycle. You can also list items you no longer want or items you're looking for.
www.reuze.co.uk

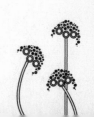

Reduce Reuse Recyle

A green guide with information on recycling facilities in your local area.

www.reducereuserecyle.co.uk

☙❧

Salvo!

This website has an online directory of antique, reclaimed, salvaged and green materials for gardens and homes.

www.salvo.co.uk

☙❧

UK FreeCycle

Helps recyclers meet to exchange items that would otherwise end up in a landfill. Check the website for your local scheme.

www.recycle4free.com

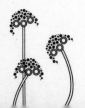

Going Green

GREEN ENERGY

The Carbon Neutral Company
Supplies carbon offset and climate change related services to business customers, and will plant trees on your behalf.
www.carbonneutral.com

The Carbon Trust
Helps business and the public sector cut carbon emissions and supports the development of low carbon technologies.
www.carbontrust.co.uk

৬৫

Ecotricity
A green electricity company that builds and invests in new, renewable energy sources like wind turbines, solar cells and hydroelectricity stations.
www.ecotricity.co.uk

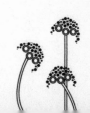

Energy Saving Trust

A non-profit making organisation that encourages energy efficiency and the integration of renewable energy sources into the economic fabric of society. The website has useful information on saving energy in the home.

www.est.org.uk

☙❧

Future London

Information on how a few simple changes can make London a greener city.

www.futurelondon.co.uk

☙❧

National Energy Foundation

Works to provide information on renewable energy and sustainable development. The website is a very useful source of information.

www.nef.org.uk/greenenergy

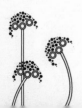

Recommended Reading

Aromatherapy Blends and Remedies, Franzesca Watson, Thorsons 1995

Ayurveda for Women, Dr Robert E. Svoboda, David & Charles 1999

The Coconut Oil Miracle, Bruce Fife, Avery Publishing 1999

A Consumer's Dictionary of Cosmetic Ingredients, Ruth Winter, Crown 1994

Dr Joshi's Holistic Detox, Dr Nish Joshi, Hodder Mobius 2006

Earl Mindell's New Vitamin Bible, Earl Mindell, Warner Books 2004

Fast Food Nation, Eric Schlosser, Penguin 2002

The Fragrant Heavens, Valerie Ann Worwood, Bantam 1999

The Fragrant Mind, Valerie Ann Worwood, Bantam 1997

The Fragrant Pharmacy, Valerie Ann Worwood, Bantam 1992

A Greener Life, Clarissa Dickson Wright and Johnny Scott, Kyle Cathie 2006

HDRA Encyclopedia of Organic Gardening, Anna Kruger, Dorling Kindersley 2005

Jamie's Dinners, Jamie Oliver, Penguin 2006

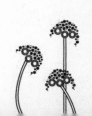

Recommended Reading

Jamie's Italy, Jamie Oliver, Michael Joseph 2005

The Naked Chef, Jamie Oliver, Penguin 2001

Not on the Label: What Really Goes into the Food on Your Plate, Felicity Lawrence, Penguin 2004

The Organic Directory 2007, Clive Litchfield 2007 (also available online on the Soil Association website)

Organic SuperFoods, Michael van Straten, Mitchell Beazley 1999

Prescription for Nutritional Healing, Phyllis Balch and James Balch, Avery Publishing 2000

Rick Stein's Food Heroes, Rick Stein, BBC Books 2005

Rick Stein's Seafood, Rick Stein, BBC Books 2006

River Café Cookbook, Rose Gray and Ruth Rogers, Ebury 1995

River Café Cookbook Book 2, Rose Gray and Ruth Rogers, Ebury 1998

The Royal Horticultural Society Organic Gardening, Pauline Pears and Sue Stickland, Mitchell Beazley 1999

The 21st Century Beauty Bible, Josephine Fairley and Sarah Stacey, Kyle Cathie 2006

Vital Oils, Liz Earle, Vermillion 2002

What's In This Stuff?: The Essential Guide to What's Really in the Products You Buy in the Supermarket, Pat Thomas, Rodale 2006

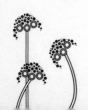

Index

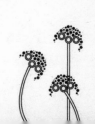

Index

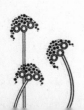

Index

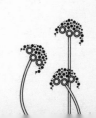

Index

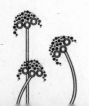

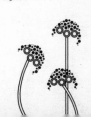

Index

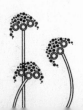

Index

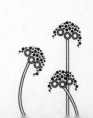

Index

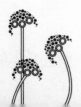